Current Clinical Strategies

Handbook of Psychiatric Drugs

1997 Edition

Donald P. Hall, Jr., M.D.

Clinical Assistant Professor of Psychiatry
Uniformed Services University of Health Sciences
Chief of Community Psychiatry
Walter Reed Army Medical Center, Washington, D.C.

Current Clinical Strategies Publishing
http://www.CCSPublishing.com

Internet Users

Visit the CCS Publishing site on the world wide web, where you can view
Current Clinical Strategies Publishing Journals on-line, and you can
view and order CCS Books:

http://www.CCSPublishing.com

Journal of Primary Care On-Line™
Journal of Medicine On-Line™
Journal of Pediatrics On-Line™
Journal of Surgery On-Line™
Journal of Family Medicine On-Line™
Journal of Emergency Medicine On-Line™
Journal of Psychiatry On-Line™
Journal of AIDS On-Line™

Obtain the most current medical information
24 hours a day

Current Clinical Strategies Publishing

27071 Cabot Road, Suite 126
Laguna Hills, California 92653
Phone: 800-331-8227
Fax: 800-965-9420
E-mail: cmcpdc234@aol.com

Printed in USA   ISBN 1-881528-15-4

Contents

Dedication

This book is dedicated to my children,
Christopher and Angela

Antidepressants

Clinical Use of Antidepressants

I. **Categories and Indications**
   A. **Tricyclic Antidepressants (TCAs)** are used in the treatment of a wide variety of psychiatric disorders, including depression, anxiety, eating disorders, and chronic pain. TCA use, however, is marked my bothersome side effects which limit patient compliance.
   B. **Serotonin Specific Reuptake Inhibitors (SSRIs)** are gradually replacing TCAs as the treatment of choice for many depressive and anxiety disorders. SSRIs have fewer side effects and are less dangerous in overdose than TCAs.
   C. **Monoamine Oxidase Inhibitors (MAOIs)**, although effective as antidepressants (especially in atypical depression), are associated with potentially hazardous side effects. MAOIs are reserved for patients who have failed trials of drugs from other categories.
   D. **Atypical Antidepressants**, which do not share the pharmacological profiles of the categories noted above, are emerging as effective agents with limited side effects (e.g., nefazodone, bupropion, and venlafaxine)

II. **Serotonin Specific Reuptake Inhibitors (SSRIs)**
   A. **SSRI Side Effects:** Gastrointestinal changes (nausea, diarrhea, abdominal pain), akathisia, diaphoresis, insomnia, anxiety, decreased appetite, weight loss, headache, dizziness, hypotension, palpitations, sexual dysfunction, lethargy, fatigue, tremor, activation of mania/hypomania, increased cholesterol, increased bleeding time, and hyponatremia.
   B. **Side Effect Management:**
      1. **GI distress** may be decreased by taking the medication 30-60 minutes after meals.
      2. **Insomnia**
         a. May be reduced by AM dosing.
         b. Trazodone (Desyrel): 25-100 mg PO qhs. Highly sedating antidepressant. Reduces primary and SSRI-induced insomnia.

      3. Sexual dysfunction:
- **a.** Decrease dose if depressive symptoms remain in remission.
- **b.** Consider changing to another agent, such as bupropion (no sexual dysfunction).

      4. Restlessness: Clonazepam (Klonopin): 0.25-0.5 mg PO bid may reduce restlessness and akathisia.

For further information on agents used to manage SSRI-induced side effects, see their individual medication listings.

C. Advantages: SSRIs have minimal adrenergic, histaminergic, and muscarinic cholinergic side effects. Therefore, they cause minimal changes in blood pressure, alertness, or mouth dryness.

D. SSRI Interactions:
1. Alcohol - Concurrent use may exacerbate depression or anxiety.
2. Antiarrhythmics - Metabolism may be impaired by SSRI.
3. Antidepressants - SSRIs may increase level of other antidepressants (e.g., tricyclic antidepressants). Levels of TCA should be checked regularly.
4. Antipsychotics - Metabolism may be impaired by SSRI. Extrapyramidal symptoms (EPS) of antipsychotics may be increased.
5. Cimetidine - May impair metabolism of SSRI.
6. Diazepam/benzodiazepines - Metabolism may be decreased by SSRI.
7. Lithium - Lithium levels may be increased.
8. MAOI - Use of MAOI within 2-4 weeks may result in serotonergic syndrome (see MAO-I section below). Concurrent use should be avoided.
9. Phenytoin, carbamazepine - Serum levels may be increased by SSRI.
10. Protein-bound drugs (e.g., warfarin, digitoxin) may be displaced by SSRI.

E. Pre-existing Medical Conditions - Use of SSRIs are not contraindicated in the presence of any medical condition.

F. Overdose - Low risk of fatality unless combined with other drugs.

III. Tricyclic Antidepressants (TCAs)

A. TCA Side Effects:
1. **Anticholinergic:** Constipation, dry mouth, blurred vision, urinary hesitancy and retention, heat intolerance, increased intraocular pressure, and tachycardia.
2. **Cardiac:** ECG changes including T-wave flattening, prolonged PR

and QT intervals, arrhythmias, and palpitations. Increased fatality risk after myocardial infarction.

   3. **Other:** Akathisia, ataxia, anxiety, agitation, memory and concentration disturbance, headache, fatigue, insomnia, nightmares, paraphasias, tremor, hematologic, agranulocytosis, anemia, ejaculatory dysfunction, and impotence.

B. **Management of TCA Side Effects**:
   1. **Sedation** may be decreased by qhs dosing after several weeks of divided dosing.
   2. **Constipation** - Stool softeners may be necessary to counteract anticholinergic effects on the bowels.
   3. **Dry mouth** may be reduced by use of hard candy and increased water consumption.

C. **Disadvantages** - TCAs are associated with greater sedation, orthostatic hypotension, and anticholinergic effects, conduction abnormalities, and risk of seizure than SSRIs.

D. **TCA Interactions:**
   1. Antihypertensives - Potentiate hypotensive side effects.
   2. Anticholinergics (e.g., antiparkinsonian agents) - Potentiate anticholinergic effects of TCAs.
   3. CNS depressants (e.g., alcohol, anticonvulsants, sedatives, antihistamines) - Potentiation of CNS depression.
   4. Disulfiram - Increases TCA level and may cause organic brain syndrome.
   5. MAOI - Contraindicated. Hypertensive crisis results (see MAOI section below).

   TCA plasma levels are increased by: Amphetamines, antipsychotics, estrogen, disulfiram, exogenous thyroid hormone, fluoxetine, glucocorticoids, oral contraceptives, salicylates, thiazides.

   TCA plasma levels are decreased by: Alcohol, barbiturates, carbamazepine, cigarettes, phenytoin, primidone, rifampin.

E. **Pre-existing Medical Conditions:**
   1. Asthma & aspirin allergy - Patients with these conditions may be more sensitive to the sulfites and tartrazine found in some TCAs, increasing the risk of allergic reaction.
   2. Conduction abnormalities - TCAs are contraindicated in patients with bifascicular block, prolonged QT interval, or left bundle branch block.
   3. Chronic pain - TCAs are often useful in the long term treatment of

pain.

4. ECT - Discontinue TCA several days prior to ECT, due to increased cardiac risks.
5. Elderly - Choose an agent with lower anticholinergic and orthostatic hypotension profile (i.e., secondary amine TCA)
6. Glaucoma - Requires concurrent use of pilocarpine.
7. Myocardial infarction - TCAs are contraindicated in the acute recovery phase due to higher mortality rate associated with type 1 antiarrhythmics.
8. Peptic ulcer disease - Antihistamine properties of doxepin may be helpful in controlling gastric acidity .
9. Pregnancy - There is little evidence of congenital malformation associated with TCAs, but use should be avoided, if possible. Use during breast feeding is discouraged.
10. Seizure disorder - TCAs lower the seizure threshold and should be avoided, if the patient has a history of seizures. Use of trazodone or Serzone should be considered in these patients.
11. Surgery - Discontinue TCA use several days before surgery to avoid drug interactions which may result in hypertension.

F. Overdose: High risk of fatality with TCA dose > 1 gram. Risk of cardiac arrhythmia for 4-5 days after overdose - may not respond to treatment. Seizures may also be difficult to control.

IV. Monamine Oxidase Inhibitors

A. MAOI Side Effects: Orthostatic hypotension, anxiety, headache, insomnia, impotence, dry mouth, agitation, dizziness, constipation, weight gain, seizures, GI distress, muscle cramps, urinary hesitancy, rash, liver damage, precipitation of mania/hypomania.

B. Monoamine Interactions:

1. Antipsychotics - May cause EPS or hypotensive reactions.
2. Meperidine - Hypotension, hypertension, fever, delirium, and death.
3. Oral hypoglycemics - Further decrease in glucose.
4. Over-the-counter cold remedies and diet pills may cause hypertensive crisis, arrhythmia, headache, convulsions.
5. Serotonergic agents (e.g., SSRIs & clomipramine) - Concurrent use may lead to a **serotonergic syndrome** (see disadvantages below).
6. TCAs, amphetamines, cocaine, anorectics, dopamine, L-dopa, methyl dopa, phenylephrine, phenylpropanolamine, norepinephrine, guanethidine, metaraminol, ephedrine, epinephrine, meperidine, other adrenergic agents, and tyramine

containing food products - Concurrent use may lead to **hypertensive crisis** (see disadvantages below).

C. **Contraindicated Dietary Factors (high tyramine content):** Canned figs, raisins, bananas, overripe fruit, fava beans (Italian green beans), sauerkraut, avocados, bean curd, soy sauce, aged yogurt, strong cheeses, sour cream, liver, spoiled meat, fermented sausages (e.g., bologna, salami, pepperoni), meat tenderizer and extracts, dried salted fish, pickled or dried herring, caviar, shrimp paste, beer, Chianti, red wine, sherry, and any non-distilled alcohol.

D. **Major Disadvantages**
   1. Risk of **serotonergic syndrome** with serotonergic agents - Manifested by anxiety, disorientation, nausea, hyperthermia, diaphoresis, autonomic instability, tremor, myoclonus, coma, and death.
   2. Risk of **hypertensive crisis** resulting from interaction with multiple medications and food groups - Manifested by headache, diaphoresis, mydriasis, hypertension, photophobia, tachycardia, bradycardia, angina, nausea/vomiting, arrhythmia, autonomic instability, renal failure, coma, and death.

E. **Treatment of Hypertensive Crisis**
   1. Recognize the symptoms.
   2. Closely monitor vital signs.
   3. Consider the use of a hypotensive agent:
      a. Nifedipine - 10 mg SL; carefully monitoring blood pressure.
      b. Phentolamine - 5 mg IV, then 0.25-0.5 mg IM q4-6 hours.
      c. Nitroprusside sodium - 0.25-10 mcg/kg/min IV; titrate dose based on blood pressure response (requires continuous blood pressure monitoring).
   4. Monitor renal function. Acidify the patient's urine. Consider dialysis in the event of significant renal impairment.
   5. Identify the cause of the crisis.

F. **Patient Instructions**
   1. Patient should notify physician before taking any medication.
   2. Wait 14 days after discontinuation of MAO-I before taking other medications.

G. **Preexisting Medical Conditions:**
   1. MAO-I use is contraindicated with cardiovascular disease, elderly (over 60), hypertension (severe), migraine headaches, renal or hepatic disease.
   2. Pregnancy - Avoid use of MAOIs due to teratogenic potential.

    H. Overdose Risks:
1. High risk of fatality, especially if combined with other drugs.
2. Seizures, arrhythmias, hypotension, or renal failure may cause death.

V. Combination Therapy for Depression
A. Indications:
1. Failure or partial response of antidepressant after trial of at least 4 weeks at recommended therapeutic dose.
2. Verified therapeutic blood level (if available) of failed therapeutic agent.

B. Augmentation: Antidepressant (e.g., TCA or SSRI) may be augmented by another agent (e.g., Lithium).
1. **Lithium:** 900-1200 mg/day, serum level 0.6-0.8 mEq/L for 7-14 day trial. Continue use if therapeutic response occurs.
2. **L-Triiodothyronine (Cytomel):** 10-50 mcg/day for 3-4 week trial. Continue if successful. Consider discontinuation of augmentation after two months.
3. **Buspirone (BuSpar):** 30-60 mg/day for 2-4 week trial. Long term use if adjunctive treatment is therapeutic.
4. **SSRI:** 20 mg/day augmentation of desipramine has been shown to be effective. Monitor serum level of TCA.

For further information on augmenting agents, see their individual medication listings.

Serotonin-Specific Reuptake Inhibitors

Fluoxetine (Prozac)

Category: SSRI
Mechanism: Inhibits presynaptic serotonin reuptake
Indications: Approved for depressive disorders and obsessive compulsive disorder. Used for other anxiety disorders (e.g., post- traumatic stress disorder, panic disorder), eating disorders (e.g., bulimia nervosa, obesity), impulse control disorders, and premenstrual dysmorphic disorder.
Preparations: 10, 20 mg tablets; 20 mg/5 ml soln.
Dosage:

> Depression - 20 mg qAM is usually effective. May increase to maximum dose of 80 mg/day. Increase dose by 20 mg/day each month if partial response.
>
> Obsessive compulsive disorder (OCD) - 20 mg/day. Increase by 20 mg/day each month if needed. Treatment of OCD tends to require higher doses than depression. Maximum dose of 80 mg/day).
>
> Panic disorder - Begin with low dose (e.g., 10 mg qAM). Increase gradually.
>
> Bulimia nervosa and obesity - 20-60 mg/day
>
> Elderly - 5-80 mg/day

Time to Therapeutic Effect: Early antidepressant effect occurs in 1-3 weeks, full effect generally requires 4-6 weeks.
Half-life: 7-9 days
Therapeutic Levels: Some suggest >200 ng/ml
Side Effect Profile: Orthostatic hypotension (low), sedation (low), anticholinergic (low), cardiac effects (low).
GI distress, insomnia, sexual dysfunction, anxiety, sedation. Also, see SSRI side effect list.
Interactions:

> **A.** Antidepressants, oral anticoagulants, and lithium levels may be increased.
>
> **B.** Highly protein bound drugs may be displaced.
>
> **C.** Diazepam may increase fluoxetine levels.
>
> **D.** Fluoxetine may impair degradation of P450 enzyme CY2D6 metabolized drugs such as TCAs, barbiturates, propranolol

antiarrhythmics, trazodone and nefazodone.

E. Also, see SSRI interaction list.

Major Safety Concern: Use of MAO-I within 5 weeks may result in serotonergic syndrome.

Contraindications: MAO-Is are contraindicated for **5 weeks** after fluoxetine. Fluoxetine is contraindicated for 2 weeks after MAO-Is.

Advantages/Disadvantages: SSRIs cause less sedation, anticholinergic effects, and postural hypotension than TCAs. No reduction of seizure threshold with SSRIs. **Long half-life** permits daily dosing and may decrease withdrawal symptoms following abrupt discontinuance of medication. Relatively safe in overdose.

Fluvoxamine (Luvox)

Category: SSRI

Mechanism: Inhibits presynaptic serotonin reuptake and potentiates norepinephrine system.

Indications: Approved for obsessive compulsive disorder. Also used clinically as antidepressant.

Preparations: 50, 100 mg tabs

Dosage:

Initially - 50 mg/day, then titrate to 300 mg/day maximum over several weeks

Elderly - 25-150 mg/day

Time to Therapeutic Effect: Early effect occurs in 1-3 weeks. Full anxiolytic effect generally occurs in 4-6 weeks.

Half-life: 16 hrs.

Therapeutic Levels: Not established

Side Effect Profile: Orthostatic hypotension (low), sedation(low), anticholinergic (low), cardiac effects (low). GI distress, insomnia, sexual dysfunction, anxiety, sedation. Also, see SSRI side effect list.

Interactions:

A. May alter level of P450 enzyme-metabolized drugs - Increasing level of TCAs, calcium channel blockers, carbamazepine, erythromycin, warfarin, phenytoin, theophylline, alprazolam, triazolam, terfenadine, propranolol.

B. Diazepam - Level both agents may be increased.

C. Also, see SSRI interaction list.

Major Safety Concern: Use of MAO-I within 2 weeks of fluvoxamine may result in serotonergic syndrome.

Contraindications: MAO-I use is contraindicated for 2 weeks before or after fluvoxamine.

Advantages/Disadvantages: SSRIs have less sedation, anticholinergic and, postural hypotension than TCAs. No reduction of seizure threshold with SSRIs. Relatively safe in overdose.

Paroxetine (Paxil)

Category: SSRI

Mechanism: Inhibits presynaptic serotonin reuptake. Also potentiates norepinephrine system.

Indications: Approved for treatment of depression, panic disorder, and obsessive compulsive disorder (OCD).

Preparations: 10, 20, 30, 40 mg tablets

Dosage:

> Initially - 10-20 mg qAM. Change to qhs dose if too sedating; may increase over several weeks (max. 50 mg/day)
>
> Depression - 20-50 mg/day
>
> Obsessive compulsive disorder - 20-60 mg/day (target of 40 mg)
>
> Panic disorder - 10-60 mg/day
>
> Elderly - 5-40 mg/day

Time to Therapeutic Effect: Early antidepressant effect occurs in 1-3 weeks. Full effect generally occurs in 4-6 weeks.

Half-life: 24 hrs.

Therapeutic Levels : Not established

Side Effect Profile: Orthostatic   hypotension (low), sedation (low), anticholinergic (moderate), cardiac effects (low). GI distress, insomnia, sexual dysfunction, anxiety, sedation. Also, see SSRI side effect list.

Interactions:

A. Diazepam - level of diazepam may be increased.

B. May increase level of highly protein bound drugs or other P450 enzyme metabolized drugs such as warfarin, phenytoin, theophylline, alprazolam triazolam, terfenadine, or propranolol.

C. Lithium level may be increased.

D. Also, see SSRI interaction list.

Major Safety Concerns: Use of MAO-I within 2 weeks may result in serotonergic syndrome. Use caution in patients with hepatic or renal disease.

Contraindications: MAO-I use is contraindicated for 2 weeks before or after paroxetine.

Advantages/Disadvantages: SSRIs have less sedation, anticholinergic, and postural hypotension than TCAs. No reduction of seizure threshold with SSRIs. Paroxetine may be less activating and more sedating than fluoxetine. **Mild anticholinergic** effects (unlike other SSRIs) may occur with paroxetine. Relatively safe in overdose.

Sertraline (Zoloft)

Category: SSRI
Mechanism: Inhibits presynaptic serotonin reuptake and potentiates dopamine.
Indications: Approved for depressive disorders. Also effective as anxiolytic (e.g., obsessive compulsive disorder, panic disorder).
Preparations: Sertraline hydrochloride: 50, 100 mg tablets
Dosage:
> Initially - 50 mg qAM, then increase to 100 mg after 3 weeks if needed (maximum dose of 200 mg/day)
> Elderly - 50-200 mg/day

Time to Therapeutic Effect: Early antidepressant effect occurs in 1-3 weeks. Full effect generally in occurs in 4-6 weeks.
Half-life: 2-4 days (includes active metabolite)
Therapeutic Levels: Not established
Side Effect Profile: Orthostatic hypotension (low), sedation (low), anticholinergic (low), cardiac effects (low). GI distress, insomnia, sexual dysfunction, anxiety, sedation. Also, see SSRI side effect list.
Interactions: Antidepressants, oral anticoagulants, lithium, some highly protein bound drugs. Also, see SSRI interaction list.
Major Safety Concern: Use of MAO-I within 2 weeks may result in serotonergic syndrome. Exercise caution in patients with renal or hepatic disease.
Contraindications: MAO-Is are contraindicated for 2 weeks before or after sertraline.
Advantages/Disadvantages: SSRIs have less sedation, anticholinergic, and postural hypotension than TCAs. No reduction of seizure threshold with SSRIs. Unlike fluoxetine, sertraline has **no significant effect on lithium** levels (monitoring lithium levels early in combination treatment, however, is still recommended). **Lowest P450 enzyme effects** of the SSRIs. Relatively safe in overdose.

Tertiary Amine Tricyclic Antidepressants

Amitriptyline (Elavil, Endep)

Category: Tertiary amine TCA

Mechanism: Inhibits presynaptic serotonin and norepinephrine reuptake.

Indications: Approved for depressive disorders. Also used for anxiety (e.g., panic disorder with agoraphobia, generalized anxiety disorder), eating disorders, and chronic pain.

Preparations: 10, 25, 50, 75, 100, 150 mg tabs; 10 mg/ml soln. (IM)

Dosage:

> Initially - 25 mg PO qhs, then increase over 2-4 week period
>
> Average dose - 150-200 mg/day
>
> Dose range - 50-300 mg/day
>
> Chronic pain syndromes - 25-100 mg qhs
>
> Elderly - 25-300 mg/day

Time to Therapeutic Effect: Early antidepressant effect occurs in 1-3 weeks. Full effect generally occurs in 4-6 weeks.

Half-life: 10-50 hrs.

Therapeutic Levels: 100-250 ng/ml (includes active metabolite)

Side Effect Profile: Orthostatic hypotension (high), sedation(high), anticholinergic (high), cardiac effects (high).Most common: sedation, dry mouth, constipation. Also, see TCA side effect list.

Interactions: No amitriptyline-specific side effects. Also, see TCA Interaction list.

Major Safety Concerns: TCAs are associated with higher rates of seizure, arrhythmia, and fatality in overdose than many other antidepressants. Use TCAs with caution in patients with a history of seizures, urinary retention, angle closure glaucoma (may require concurrent medication treatment), cardiovascular disease, or stroke.

Contraindications: Use of TCAs is contraindicated in the acute recovery phase following myocardial infarction due to increased risk of fatal arrhythmia. MAO-I use is contraindicated for 2 weeks before or after TCAs due to risk of hypertensive crisis.

Advantages/Disadvantages: Amitriptyline is widely used in the treatment of **chronic pain**. Sedative quality of TCA may be useful in the treatment of depression associated with significant insomnia or anxiety. TCAs (especially tertiary amines) are associated with greater incidence of unwanted side effects and lethality in overdose than SSRIs.

Clomipramine (Anafranil)

Category: Tertiary amine TCA
Mechanism: Inhibits presynaptic serotonin reuptake and potentiates dopamine.
Indications: Approved for **obsessive compulsive disorder** (OCD). Also used for treatment of depression and other anxiety disorders (e.g., panic disorder with agoraphobia).
Preparations: 25, 50, 75 mg caps
Dosage:
> Initially - 25 mg qhs, then increase over 2-4 week period
> Average dose - 150-200 mg/day
> Range of dosing - 50-250 mg/day
> Panic disorder - 25-75 mg qhs

Time to Therapeutic Effect: Early antidepressant/anxiolytic effects occur in 1-3 weeks, full effect generally occurs in 4-6 weeks. OCD symptoms may take longer to respond (1-3 months).
Half-life: 20-50 hrs.
Therapeutic Levels: 150-300 ng/ml
Side Effect Profile: Orthostatic hypotension (high), sedation(high), anticholinergic (high), cardiac effects (high). Shares side effects of SSRI category (see SSRI side effect list) and TCA category (see TCA side effect list).
Interactions: Avoid concurrent use of drugs which lower seizure threshold. Also, see TCA interaction list.
Major Safety Concerns: TCAs are associated with higher rates of seizure, arrhythmia, and fatality in overdose than many other antidepressants. Use TCAs with caution in patients with a history of seizures, urinary retention, angle closure glaucoma (may require concurrent medication treatment), cardiovascular disease, or stroke.
Contraindications: Use of TCAs is contraindicated in the acute recovery phase following myocardial infarction due to increased risk of fatal arrhythmia. MAO-I use is contraindicated for 2 weeks before or after TCAs due to risk of hypertensive crisis.
Advantages/Disadvantages: Clomipramine may be especially useful in depressed patients with strong obsessional features. Sedative quality of TCA may be useful in the treatment of depression associated with significant

insomnia or anxiety. TCAs (especially tertiary amines) are associated with greater incidence of unwanted side effects and lethality in overdose than SSRIs. Clomipramine has higher risk of **seizures** than other TCAs.

Doxepin (Adapin, Sinequan)

Category: Tertiary amine TCA
Mechanism: Inhibits serotonin and norepinephrine reuptake
Indications: Depressive disorders. Used clinically to treat anxiety and chronic pain disorders
Preparations: 15, 25, 50, 75, 100, 150 mg tablets; 10 mg/ml conc. (PO)
Dosage:
  Initially: 25 mg qhs or bid, then increase over 2-4 week period
  Average dose: 150-200 mg/day
  Dose range: 25-300 mg/day
  Elderly: 15-300 mg/day
Half-Life: 8-24 hrs.
Therapeutic Levels: 100-250 ng/ml
Time to Therapeutic Effect: Early antidepressant effect occurs in 1-3 weeks. Full effect generally occurs in 4-6 weeks
Side Effect Profile: Orthostatic hypotension (high), sedation (high), anticholinergic (moderate), cardiac effects (moderate). Most common: sedation, dry mouth, constipation. Also, see TCA side effect list.
Interactions: More likely than other TCAs to potentiate sedating effects of other medications. Also, see TCA interaction list.
Major Safety Concerns: TCAs are associated with higher rates of seizure, arrhythmia, and fatality in overdose than many other antidepressants. Use TCAs with caution in patients with a history of seizures, urinary retention, angle closure glaucoma (may require concurrent medication treatment), cardiovascular disease, or stroke.
Contraindications: Use of TCAs is contraindicated in the acute recovery phase following myocardial infarction due to increased risk of fatal arrhythmia. MAO-I use is contraindicated for 2 weeks before or after TCAs due to risk of hypertensive crisis.
Advantages/Disadvantages: Doxepin is often used in the treatment of **chronic pain**. It is the **most sedating TCA**. This sedative quality may be useful in the treatment of depression associated with significant insomnia or anxiety. Doxepin's strong antihistamine (H2) properties may be useful in the management of **peptic ulcer disease**. TCAs (especially tertiary amines) are associated with greater incidence of unwanted side effects and lethality in

overdose than SSRIs.

Imipramine (Tofranil)

Category: Tertiary amine TCA
Mechanism: Inhibits serotonin and norepinephrine reuptake
Indications: Depressive disorders. Clinically used to treat anxiety disorders (e.g., panic disorder), anorexia and bulimia, chronic pain, and enuresis.
Preparations:
Imipramine hydrochloride - 10, 25, 50 mg tabs; 12.5 mg/ml soln. (IM)
Imipramine pamoate - 75, 100, 125, 150 mg caps
Dosage:
    Initially: 25 mg qhs, then increase over 2-4 week period
    Average dose: 150-200 mg/day
    Dose range: 50-300 mg/day
    Elderly: 30-40 mg qhs (max. 200 mg/day)
Half-Life: 5-25 hrs.
Therapeutic Levels: 150-300 ng/ml
Time to Therapeutic Effect: Early antidepressant effect occurs in 1-3 weeks. Full effect generally occurs in 4-6 weeks.
Side Effect Profile: Orthostatic hypotension (high), sedation (high), anticholinergic (high), cardiac effects (high). Most common: sedation, dry mouth, constipation. Also, see TCA side effect list.
Interactions: No imipramine-specific interactions. See TCA interaction list.
Major Safety Concerns: TCAs are associated with higher rates of seizure, arrhythmia, and fatality in overdose than many other antidepressants. Use TCAs with caution in patients with a history of seizures, urinary retention, angle closure glaucoma (may require concurrent medication treatment), cardiovascular disease, or stroke.
Contraindications: Use of TCAs is contraindicated in the acute recovery phase following myocardial infarction due to increased risk of fatal arrhythmia. MAO-I use is contraindicated for 2 weeks before or after TCAs due to risk of hypertensive crisis.
Advantages/Disadvantages: Imipramine has well documented effectiveness in the treatment of **panic disorder**. Sedative quality of TCA may be useful in the treatment of depression associated with significant insomnia or anxiety. TCAs (especially tertiary amines) are associated with greater incidence of unwanted side effects and lethality in overdose than SSRIs.

Trimipramine (Surmontil)

Category: Tertiary amine TCA
Mechanism: Inhibits serotonin and norepinephrine reuptake
Indications: Depressive disorders
Preparations: 25, 50, 100 mg caps
Dosage:
    Initially: 25 mg qhs, then increase over 2-4 week period.
    Average dose: 150-200 mg/day
    Range of doses: 50-300 mg/day
    Elderly: 25-50 mg qhs (max. 200 mg/day)
Therapeutic Levels: Unknown
Time to Therapeutic Effect: Early antidepressant effect occurs in 1-3 weeks. Full effect generally occurs in 4-6 weeks.
Side Effect Profile: Orthostatic hypotension (high), sedation (high), anticholinergic (high), cardiac effects (high).Most common: sedation, dry mouth, constipation. Also, see TCA side effect list.
Interactions: No trimipramine-specific interactions. See TCA interaction list.
Major Safety Concerns: TCAs are associated with higher rates of seizure, arrhythmia, and fatality in overdose than many other antidepressants. Use TCAs with caution in patients with a history of seizures, urinary retention, angle closure glaucoma (may require concurrent medication treatment), cardiovascular disease, or stroke.
Contraindications: Use of TCAs is contraindicated in the acute recovery phase following myocardial infarction due to increased risk of fatal arrhythmia. MAO-I use is contraindicated for 2 weeks before or after TCAs due to risk of hypertensive crisis.
Advantages/Disadvantages: Sedative quality of TCA may be useful in the treatment of depression associated with significant insomnia or anxiety. TCAs (especially tertiary amines) are associated with greater incidence of unwanted side effects and lethality in overdose than SSRIs.

Secondary Amine Tricyclic Antidepressants

Desipramine (Norpramin)

Category: Secondary amine TCA

Mechanism: Inhibits serotonin and norepinephrine reuptake

Indications: Depressive disorders. Clinically used to treat anxiety, anorexia, bulimia, and chronic pain disorders.

Preparations: 10, 25, 50, 75, 100, 150 mg tabs

Dosage:

    Initially: 25 mg qhs, then increase over 2-4 week period

    Average dose: 150-200 mg/day

    Dose range: 50-300 mg/day

    Elderly: 25-100 mg/day (max. 200 mg/day)

Half-Life: 12-24 hrs.

Therapeutic Levels: 125-300 ng/ml

Time to Therapeutic Effect: Early antidepressant effect occurs in 1-3 weeks. Full effect generally occurs in 4-6 weeks.

Side Effect Profile: Orthostatic hypotension (high), sedation (moderate), anticholinergic (moderate), cardiac effects (moderate). Most common: sedation, dry mouth, constipation. Also, see TCA side effect list.

Interactions: No desipramine-specific interactions. See TCA interaction list.

Major Safety Concerns: TCAs are associated with higher rates of seizure, arrhythmia, and fatality in overdose than many other antidepressants. Use TCAs with caution in patients with a history of seizures, urinary retention, angle closure glaucoma (may require concurrent medication treatment), cardiovascular disease, or stroke.

Contraindications: Use of TCAs is contraindicated in the acute recovery phase following myocardial infarction due to increased risk of fatal arrhythmia. MAO-I use is contraindicated for 2 weeks before or after TCAs due to risk of hypertensive crisis.

Advantages/Disadvantages: Desipramine is **among the least sedating and least anticholinergic TCAs**. TCAs are associated with greater incidence of unwanted side effects and lethality in overdose than SSRIs. Secondary amines, however, have less side effects than tertiary amines.

Nortriptyline (Pamelor, Aventyl)

Category: Secondary amine TCA
Mechanism: Inhibits serotonin, norepinephrine and, dopamine reuptake.
Indications: Depressive disorders. Clinically used to treat anxiety and chronic pain disorders.
Preparations: 10, 25, 50, 75 mg capsules; 10 mg/5 ml soln. (PO)
Dosage:
    Initially: 25 mg qhs, then increase over 2-4 week period
    Average dose: 75-150 mg/day
    Dose range: 25-150 mg/day
    Elderly: 10-75 mg/day (max. 150 mg/day)
Half-Life: 18-44 hrs.
Therapeutic Levels: 50-160 ng/ml
Time to Therapeutic Effect: Early antidepressant effect in 1-3 weeks, full effect generally in 4-6 weeks.
Side Effect Profile: Orthostatic hypotension (low), sedation (moderate), anticholinergic (moderate), cardiac effects (moderate). Most common: sedation, dry mouth, constipation. Also, see TCA side effect list.
Interactions: See TCA Interaction list.
Major Safety Concerns: TCAs are associated with higher rates of seizure, arrhythmia, and fatality in overdose than many other antidepressants. Use TCAs with caution in patients with a history of seizures, urinary retention, angle closure glaucoma (may require concurrent medication treatment), cardiovascular disease, or stroke.
Contraindications: Use of TCAs is contraindicated in the acute recovery phase following myocardial infarction due to increased risk of fatal arrhythmia. MAO-I use is contraindicated for 2 weeks before or after TCAs due to risk of hypertensive crisis.
Advantages/Disadvantages: Desipramine is widely used in the treatment of **chronic pain**. It is **among the least likely TCAs to cause orthostatic hypotension**. TCAs are associated with greater incidence of unwanted side effects and lethality in overdose than SSRIs. Secondary amines, however, have less side effects than tertiary amines.

Protriptyline (Vivactil)

Category: Secondary amine TCA

Mechanism: Inhibits serotonin and norepinephrine reuptake

Indications: Depressive disorders

Preparations: 5, 10 mg tabs

Dosage:

> Initially: 5 mg qAM, then increase over 2 weeks period. No doses within 3 hours of bedtime.
> Average dose: 15-40 mg/day
> Dose range: 10-60 mg/day
> Elderly: 5 mg tid (max. 40 mg/day)

Half-Life: 50-200 hrs.

Therapeutic Levels: 75-200 ng/ml

Time to Therapeutic Effect: Early antidepressant effect in 1-3 weeks, full effect generally in 4-6 weeks.

Side Effect Profile: Orthostatic hypotension (moderate), sedation (low), anticholinergic (moderate), cardiac effects (high). Also, see TCA side effect list.

Interactions: No protriptyline-specific interactions. See TCA interaction list.

Major Safety Concerns: TCAs are associated with higher rates of seizure, arrhythmia, and fatality in overdose than many other antidepressants. Use TCAs with caution in patients with a history of seizures, urinary retention, angle closure glaucoma (may require concurrent medication treatment), cardiovascular disease, or stroke.

Contraindications: Use of TCAs is contraindicated in the acute recovery phase following myocardial infarction due to increased risk of fatal arrhythmia. MAO-I use is contraindicated for 2 weeks before or after TCAs due to risk of hypertensive crisis.

Advantages/Disadvantages: Protriptyline is the **least sedating and most activating TCA**. TCAs are associated with greater incidence of unwanted side effects and lethality in overdose than SSRIs. Secondary amines, however, have less side effects than tertiary amines.

Tetracyclic Antidepressants

Amoxapine (Asendin)

Category: Tetracyclic antidepressant
Mechanism: Inhibits norepinephrine (primarily) and serotonin reuptake. Dopamine antagonist effects by metabolite (loxapine).
Indications: Depressive disorders. Some clinicians prefer use of this drug in depression with psychotic features.
Preparations: 25, 50, 100, 150 mg tabs
Dosage:
  Initially: 50 mg PO qhs , then increase over 1-3 week period to 100 mg bid/tid
  Average dose: 200-250 mg/day
  Dose range: 50-300 mg/day
  Elderly: Start with 25 mg qhs; increase to 50 mg bid/tid (max. 300 mg/day)
Half-Life: 8 hrs.
Therapeutic Levels: 100-250 ng/ml
Time to Therapeutic Effect: Early antidepressant effect occurs in 1-3 weeks. Full effect generally occurs in 4-6 weeks.
Side Effect Profile: Orthostatic hypotension (low), sedation (moderate), anticholinergic (high), cardiac effects (high).Possible extrapyramidal symptoms (EPS) due to dopamine antagonism of loxapine (e.g., dystonia, akinesia, Parkinsonian symptoms), urinary retention, constipation, dry mouth, blurred vision, insomnia, sedation, CNS stimulation, seizure, GI upset, weight gain, hypotension, rash. Shares side effects of TCAs and dopamine antagonists. Also, see TCA and antipsychotic side effect lists.
Interactions: Interactions include both TCA and dopamine antagonist profiles. See TCA and antipsychotic interaction lists.
Major Safety Concerns: Tardive dyskinesia and neuroleptic malignant syndrome are possible due to dopamine antagonist side effects. Amoxapine is associated with higher rates of seizure, arrhythmia, and fatality in overdose than many other antidepressants. Use amoxapine with caution in patients with a history of seizures, urinary retention, angle closure glaucoma (may require concurrent medication treatment), cardiovascular disease, or stroke.
Contraindications: Use of amoxapine is contraindicated in the acute recovery phase following myocardial infarction due to increased risk of fatal arrhythmia. MAO-I use is contraindicated for 2 weeks before or after amoxapine due to risk of hypertensive crisis.

Advantages/Disadvantages: Amoxapine is metabolized to loxapine (dopamine antagonist). The antipsychotic properties of loxapine may be useful in the treatment of psychotic features in a depressed patient. The added risk of dopamine antagonist side effects such as **tardive dyskinesia**, however, may expose the patient to unnecessary side effects in long term treatment. Use of separate antidepressant and antipsychotic is recommended.

Maprotiline (Ludiomil)

Category: Tetracyclic antidepressant
Mechanism: Inhibits norepinephrine reuptake
Indications: Depressive disorders
Preparations: 25, 50, 75 mg tabs
Dosage:
> Initially: 75 mg qhs for 2 weeks, then increase in 25 mg increments over 3-4 week period. Use divided doses.
> Average dose: 100-150 mg/day
> Dose range: 50-200 mg/day
> Elderly: Start with 25 mg qhs. Increase to 50-75 qhs (max. 100 mg/day)

Half-Life: 21-25 hrs.
Therapeutic Levels: 150-300 ng/ml
Time to Therapeutic Effect: Early antidepressant effect occurs in 1-3 weeks. Full effect generally occurs in 4-6 weeks
Side Effect Profile: Orthostatic hypotension (moderate), sedation (moderate), anticholinergic (moderate), cardiac effects (moderate). Drowsiness, headache, CNS stimulation, seizure, photosensitivity, nausea, fatigue, rash. Similar to TCA profile. See TCA side effect list.
Interactions: Avoid medications which lower seizure threshold. Similar to TCA profile. See TCA interaction list.
Major Safety Concern: Avoid use of maprotiline in patients with risk of alcohol or benzodiazepine withdrawal syndrome. Maprotiline is associated with higher rates of seizure, arrhythmia, and fatality in overdose than many other antidepressants. Use maprotiline with caution in patients with a history of seizures, urinary retention, angle closure glaucoma (may require concurrent medication treatment), cardiovascular disease, or stroke.
Contraindications: Use of maprotiline is contraindicated in the acute recovery phase following myocardial infarction due to increased risk of fatal arrhythmia. MAO-I use is contraindicated for 2 weeks before or after maprotiline due to risk of hypertensive crisis.
Advantages/Disadvantages: Maprotiline is associated with a higher risk of

seizure than most other antidepressants. Its long half life may necessitate longer period of observation after overdose.

Monoamine Oxidase Inhibitors

Phenelzine (Nardil)

Category: MAO-I
Mechanism: Inhibits monoamine degradation in the synapse.
Indications: Approved for atypical depression. Also used clinically for anxiety disorders such as panic disorder with agoraphobia. Not recommended as first line treatment.
Preparations: 15 mg tabs
Dosage:
> Initial dosing: 15 mg bid; increase by 15 mg/day each week
> Average doses: 30-60 mg/day
> Dose range: 15-90 mg/day
> Elderly: Start with 7.5-15 mg/day; max. 60 mg/day

Therapeutic Levels: Not established. Some clinical investigators measure platelet MAO-I activity. Therapeutic effect is associated with >80% inhibition of platelet activity.
Time to Antidepressant Effect: 3-6 weeks
Side Effect Profile: Orthostatic hypotension (high), sedation (moderate), anticholinergic (low), cardiac effects (moderate). Most frequent: Orthostatic hypotension, edema, insomnia, weight gain, sexual dysfunction. Pyridoxine deficiency may develop. Also, see MAO-I side effect list.
Interactions: Numerous medication (e.g., sympathomimetics) and dietary (i.e., tyramine) interactions. See MAO-I interaction list.
Contraindications: Do not use MAO-Is in elderly patients (over 60 years) or in those with a history of pheochromocytoma, liver disease or abnormal LFTs, cardiovascular disease, hypertension (severe), migraine headaches, or renal disease. Concurrent or rapid succession use of other MAO-I or other antidepressants is contraindicated. Elective surgery involving general anesthesia is contraindicated during MAO-I use. Discontinue MAO-I 10 days prior to surgery. **Meperidine** interaction has been associated with fatality. Avoid **tyramine** containing foods. An extensive list of contraindicated medications and dietary factors is presented in the MAO-I general principles section.
Major Safety Concerns: **Hypertensive crisis** is possible with numerous medication interactions. High fatality risk is associated with MAO-I overdose. Fatal hepatic damage rarely occurs (monitor LFTs). Avoid MAOIs during pregnancy (MAOIs are teratogenic).

Advantages/Disadvantages: Major morbidity and mortality risks are associated with MAO-I use. Phenelzine is associated with a higher incidence of weight gain, drowsiness, dry mouth, and sexual dysfunction than tranylcypromine.

Tranylcypromine (Parnate)

Category: MAO-I
Mechanism: Inhibits monoamine degradation in synapse
Indications: Approved for atypical depression. Also used clinically for anxiety disorders such as panic disorder with agoraphobia. Not recommended as first line treatment.
Preparations: 10 mg tabs
Dosage:
> Initial dosing: 10 mg bid. Increase by 10 mg/day each week.
> Average dose: 20-40 mg/day
> Dose range: 10-60 mg/day
> Elderly: Start with 5-10 mg/day; max. 30-40 mg/day

Therapeutic Levels: Not established. Some clinical investigators measure platelet MAO-I activity. Therapeutic effect is associated with >80% inhibition of platelet activity.
Time to Antidepressant Effect: 3-6 weeks
Side Effect Profile: Orthostatic hypotension (high), sedation (moderate), anticholinergic (low), cardiac effects (moderate). Most frequent: Orthostatic hypotension, edema, insomnia, weight gain, sexual dysfunction. Pyridoxine deficiency may develop. Also, see MAO-I side effect list.
Interactions: Numerous medication (e.g., sympathomimetics) and dietary (i.e., tyramine) interactions. See MAO-I interaction list.
Contraindications: Do not use MAO-Is in elderly patients (over 60 years) or those with a history of pheochromocytoma, liver disease or abnormal LFTs, cardiovascular disease, hypertension (severe), migraine headaches, or renal disease. Concurrent or rapid succession use of other MAO-I or other antidepressant is contraindicated. Elective surgery involving general anesthesia is contraindicated during MAO-I use. Discontinue MAO-I 10 days prior to surgery. **Meperidine** interaction has been associated with fatality. Avoid **tyramine** containing foods. An extensive list of contraindicated medications and dietary factors is presented in the MAO-I general principles section.
Major Safety Concerns: Hypertensive crisis is possible with numerous medication interactions. High fatality risk is associated with MAO-I overdose.

Fatal hepatic damage rarely occurs (monitor LFTs). Avoid MAOIs during pregnancy (MAOIs found to be teratogenic in animal studies)

Advantages/Disadvantages: Major morbidity and mortality risks are associated with MAO-I use. Phenelzine is associated with higher incidences of weight gain, drowsiness, dry mouth, and sexual dysfunction than tranylcypromine.

Atypical Antidepressants

Bupropion (Wellbutrin)

Category: Unicyclic antidepressant
Mechanism: Inhibits norepinephrine reuptake
Indications: Approved for depressive disorders. Also used clinically for attention deficit/hyperactivity disorder.
Preparations: 75, 100 mg tabs
Dosage:

Initially: 100 mg bid, then increase to 100 tid after 4-5 days
Do not increase greater than 100 mg within 3 days.
Average dose: 300 mg/day (divided doses)
Do not exceed 150 mg/dose.
Dose range: 75-450 mg/day (max. 450 mg/day)
Elderly: 75-450 mg/day

Half-Life: 4-24 hrs.
Therapeutic Levels: Not established. Some suggest 10-60 mcg/ml
Time to Therapeutic Effect: Early antidepressant effect occurs in 1-3 weeks. Full effect generally occurs in 4-6 weeks.
Side Effect Profile: Orthostatic hypotension (low), sedation (low), anticholinergic (low), cardiac effects (low). Most common: insomnia, CNS stimulation, headache, constipation, dry mouth, nausea, tremor, seizure.
Interactions: May interact with hepatically metabolized medications (e.g., carbamazepine, cimetidine, barbiturates, phenytoin).Dopamine agonists may lead to confusion, dyskinesia, seizure. Also, see contraindications.
Major Safety Concern: Use caution in patients with hepatic, renal, or cardiac disease. Bupropion is not recommend during pregnancy or lactation. Monitor LFTs for hepatotoxicity.
Seizure risk: Early clinical research suggested that bupropion had a seizure rate of 0.4% (4 times higher than most antidepressants) at doses less than 450 mg/day and 4% at doses of 450-600 mg/day. Recent clinical studies, however, suggest that the seizure rate is equal to that of other antidepressants at doses up to 450 mg/day.
Contraindications: Bupropion is contraindicated for 2 weeks before or after MAO-I. Avoid bupropion use in patients with anorexia or bulimia, due to possible electrolyte changes potentiating seizure. Do not use bupropion in patients with a history of seizure, brain injury or EEG abnormality, or recent history of alcohol withdrawal. Avoid medications which lower seizure threshold

(e.g., other antidepressants, lithium).

Advantages/Disadvantages: Bupropion has fewer side effects than TCAs and less sexual dysfunction than SSRIs. It is not associated with orthostatic hypotension or weight gain. Bupropion may be useful in patients with cardiovascular disease due to minimal associated changes in ventricular function or cardiac conduction. Bupropion has a greater risk of **seizure at doses above 450 mg/day** than most TCAs. A new sustained release form, currently under investigation, will lower the risk of seizure.

Nefazodone (Serzone)

Category: Phenylpiperazine analog of trazodone

Mechanism: Inhibits presynaptic serotonin reuptake and blocks postsynaptic serotonin-2 receptors

Indications: Approved for depressive disorders. Used clinically for premenstrual dysphoric disorder and chronic pain.

Preparations: 100, 150, 200, 250 mg tabs

Dosage:
> Initially: 50 qd - 100 bid, then increase gradually after 1 week as needed
> Average dose: 300-500 mg/day (bid doses)
> Dose range: 50-600 mg/day
> Elderly: start with 50 mg/day, range: 100-200 bid

Half-Life: 2-4 hrs.; metabolite 2-18 hrs.

Therapeutic Levels: Not established

Time to Therapeutic Effect: Early antidepressant effect occurs in 1-3 weeks. Full effect generally occurs in 4-6 weeks.

Side Effects: Orthostatic hypotension (low), sedation (low), anticholinergic (low), cardiac effects (low). Most common: nausea, dry mouth, dizziness, sedation, agitation, constipation, postural hypotension, and headache.

Interactions: Levels of triazolam and alprazolam may be increased. Also, see contraindications.

Major Safety Concern: Concurrent MAO-I use may cause serotonergic syndrome (see MAO-I section). Clearance is reduced in elderly patients and those with hepatic impairment.

Contraindications: Nefazodone is contraindicated for 2 weeks before or after MAO-I. Do not use nefazodone with astemizole (Hismanal) or terfenadine (Seldane).

Advantages/Disadvantages: Unlike most other antidepressants, nefazodone causes **minimal suppression of REM sleep**. It is associated with fewer side effects than TCAs or trazodone. **No sexual dysfunction** has been noted with nefazodone. It reduces depression related anxiety and agitation. Nefazodone does not have the alpha adrenergic or histamine antagonism effects seen with trazodone.

Trazodone (Desyrel)

Category: Triazolopyridine

Mechanism: Inhibits presynaptic serotonin reuptake. Some postsynaptic serotonin agonist effects by metabolite.

Indications: Approved for depressive disorders. Used clinically for insomnia, anxiety; and agitation in the elderly.

Preparations: 50, 100, 150, 300 mg tabs

Dosage:

    Initially: 50 mg qhs, then increase by 50 mg/day as tolerated (divided doses)

    Average dose: 300-600 mg/day

    Dose range: 200-600 mg/day

    Elderly: 50-500 mg/day

    Insomnia: 25-100 qhs

Half-Life: 4-9 hrs.

Therapeutic Levels: 800-1600 ng/mcL

Time to Therapeutic Effect: Early antidepressant effect occurs in 1-3 weeks. Full effect generally occurs in 4-6 weeks.

Side Effect Profile: Orthostatic hypotension (moderate), sedation (high), anticholinergic (low), cardiac effects (moderate). Most common: drowsiness, dizziness, GI irritation, fatigue, CNS stimulation, headache, nausea, dry mouth, blurred vision, hypotension, syncope, sexual dysfunction, **priapism** - rare (treatment may include Intracavernosal injection of epinephrine in emergency situation).

Interactions: Trazodone may potentiate CNS depressants and antihypertensives. Fluoxetine may increase level of trazodone. Trazodone may alter level and function of anticoagulants.

Major Safety Concern: Avoid use of trazodone during ETC. Exercise great caution when combining trazodone with an MAO-I.

Contraindications: Trazodone is contraindicated in the acute recovery phase following myocardial infarction. Avoid use of trazodone in pregnancy and lactation (teratogenic in animals), and in patients with a history of ventricular arrhythmia.

Advantages/Disadvantages: Sedating side effects of low dose trazodone are useful in **treatment of insomnia with or without associated depression**.

Trazodone has minor cardiac side effects and is less fatal in overdose than TCAs. Trazodone's short half life warrants bid dosing.

Venlafaxine (Effexor)

Category: Phenylethylamine
Mechanism: Inhibits reuptake of serotonin and norepinephrine.
Indications: Approved for depressive disorders. May be useful clinically for attention deficit/hyperactivity disorder (ADHD) and chronic pain.
Preparations: 25, 37.5, 50, 75, 100 mg tabs
Dosage:

> Initially: 25 mg qd on first day , then 25 mg PO tid. Increase as tolerated to 50 mg tid. Do not increase more than 75 mg/day within a 4 day interval. After 3-4 weeks), dose may be decreased if symptoms remain in remission. Some patients are maintained on 75 mg/day.
> Average dose: 75-250 mg/day
> Dose range: 75-375 mg/day (divided doses)
> Elderly: 75-375 mg/day

Half-Life: 5 hrs.
Therapeutic Levels: Not established
Time to Therapeutic Effect: Antidepressant effect occurs in 1-3 weeks.
Side Effect Profile: Orthostatic hypotension (low), sedation (low), anticholinergic (low), cardiac effects (low). Most common: nausea, insomnia, sedation, dry mouth, constipation, dizziness, anxiety, decreased appetite, blurred vision, sexual dysfunction, elevated blood pressure with doses above 300 mg/day (generally, elevations are clinically insignificant in otherwise healthy adults).
Interactions: Levels may be altered by hepatically metabolized agent (e.g., cimetidine). No evidence of interaction with diazepam or lithium. May potentiate sympathomimetics.
Major Safety Concern: Decrease dose by ½ in patients with significant renal or hepatic disease.
Contraindications: MAO-I use is contraindicated for 2 weeks before or after venlafaxine.
Advantages/Disadvantages: Venlafaxine may have a faster antidepressant effect than other agents and may be more effective in the treatment of melancholic depression. Its short half life makes bid/tid dosing necessary. Venlafaxine requires tapering to discontinue use.

Antipsychotics

Clinical Use of Antipsychotics

I. **Categories and Indications:** Antipsychotics may be divided into two primary categories: **Typical and atypical agents**. Both groups are indicated for the treatment of psychosis and severe agitation. Typical antipsychotic agents have been, historically, the first-line treatment for thought disorder. New atypical antipsychotics, however, are challenging this first-line position because of their greater efficacy and lesser side effect concerns. Only three atypical agents are currently available: Clozapine (Clozaril), olanzapine (Zyprexa) and risperidone (Risperdal).

II. **Pharmacology:** Typical and atypical antipsychotics are distinguished primarily by their antagonist effects on the dopamine-2 (D2) receptor system.
    A. **Typical antipsychotic agents** possess **high affinity for D2** receptors.
        1. Typical antipsychotic agents may be divided into high, moderate, and low potency categories based on their level of dopamine receptor antagonism.
        2. All agents within the typical antipsychotic category are equally effective, but vary in the amounts of drug required to block D2 receptors and elicit antipsychotic activity.
            a. High potency agents have the highest affinity for D2 receptors and require the lowest amounts of drug to exert an antipsychotic effect.
            b. Low potency agents have lower D2 affinity and require larger doses of drug to elicit an antipsychotic effect.
    B. **Atypical agents** have **relatively low affinity for D2** receptors. Pharmacologic mechanisms for their antipsychotic effects are unknown. Multiple neurotransmitter systems are effected.
        1. Olanzapine is an antagonist of serotonin-2, alpha-1 adrenergic, and dopamine-2 receptors.
        2. Risperidone is an antagonist of serotonin, alpha-adrenergic, and dopamine-2 receptors.
        3. Clozapine is an antagonist of serotonin, alpha-adrenergic, and dopamine-1,2,&4 receptors. Clozapine also possesses significant anti-histamine and anti-cholinergic properties leading to a side effect profile similar to that of the typical low potency agents.

III. Efficacy

A. **Positive symptoms:** No differences have been clearly proven in the efficacy of typical and atypical agents in the treatment of the positive symptoms (e.g., hallucinations) of new-onset thought disorders.

B. **Negative symptoms:** Atypical agents are more effective in the treatment of the negative symptoms (e.g., blunted affect and poor motivation) of schizophrenia.

C. **Treatment resistant psychosis:** Patients failing to respond to drug trials of 1-2 typical agents may respond to an atypical agent. Clozapine use leads to significant improvement in 30% of patients who have done poorly on typical agents. Further research is needed to determine benefits of risperidone and olanzapine.

IV. Morbidity

A. **Tardive dyskinesia (TD)** is a long term, often permanent, neurological impairment resulting from extensive use of typical antipsychotics. **Atypical agents, however, have minimal associated risk of TD**.

B. **Neuroleptic malignant syndrome** is an uncommon, yet potentially fatal, adverse reaction to typical antipsychotics. Although some risk of Neuroleptic malignant syndrome is present with risperidone use, this risk is minimal with clozapine.

V. Choosing an Antipsychotic Agent: Choice of an antipsychotic agent is typically guided by the patient's history of response to medication and the side effect profile of the antipsychotic.

A. For **new onset psychosis**, most clinicians begin with a typical agent. Specific agents may be chosen based on desired sedative or anticholinergic side effects. Sedative effects are useful in agitated patients. Anticholinergic effects are useful in the control of extrapyramidal symptoms.

B. For patients with a history of **poor response of positive symptoms** to adequate medication trials with two typical agents, an atypical agent should be considered.
1. Clozapine has proven effectiveness in the management of treatment refractory patients.
2. Risperidone and olanzapine may be more effective for patients who are refractory to other agents, but only limited data are available.

C. **Poor response of negative symptoms** is another indication for trial of an atypical agent. All three atypical agents have greater efficacy than typical agents in treatment of the negative symptoms of schizophrenia.

D. Patients with **tardive dyskinesia (TD)** should be considered for treatment with an atypical agent to avoid progression of neurological impairment.

1. Clozapine is not associated with TD.
2. Risperidone is associated with a minimal incidence of TD.
3. Olanzapine (Zyprexa) is expected to have minimal associated risk of TD.

VI. Pharmacokinetics

A. After oral absorption, peak plasma levels of antipsychotics usually occur within 2-4 hours. Liquid preparations are absorbed more quickly. IM injections reach peak levels in 30-60 minutes.

B. Antipsychotic agents undergo extensive hepatic conjugation. 50% of the antipsychotic is excreted via enterohepatic circulation and 50% through the kidneys.

C. Antipsychotics are 85-90% protein bound and highly lipophilic.

D. Half-lives generally range from 15-50 hours. Steady plasma levels may take 5-10 days to establish.

VII. **Side Effect Pharmacology:** In general, low potency typical antipsychotic agents have more troublesome side effects than high potency agents due to greater antagonism of cholinergic, adrenergic, and histaminergic receptors. High potency agents, however, have more frequent extrapyramidal side effects due to potent antagonism of dopamine receptors.

Although these distinctions are useful, all agents within the typical antipsychotic category share some risk of each type of side effect. Side effect profiles resulting from antagonism of these receptor systems may be summarized as follows:

A. **Muscarinic cholinergic** side effects - dry mouth, constipation, urine retention, blurred vision, precipitation of narrow angle glaucoma.

B. **Alpha-1 adrenergic** side effects - orthostatic hypotension, static hypotension, lightheadedness, tachycardia, sedation.

C. **Histamine-1** side effects - sedation, weight gain.

D. **Dopamine-2** side effects- extrapyramidal symptoms (e.g., dystonic reactions, masked facies, shuffling gait); not present with clozapine.

VIII. **Antipsychotic Side Effects:** Drug-induced Parkinsonism (masked facies, shuffling gait, fine tremor), tardive dyskinesia, neuroleptic malignant syndrome, dystonic reaction, akathisia (restlessness), prolactin elevation, galactorrhea, amenorrhea, sexual dysfunction, fatigue, blurred vision, precipitation of narrow angle glaucoma, dry mouth, constipation, urine retention, orthostatic hypotension, static hypotension, lightheadedness, tachycardia, sedation, weight gain, hyperthermia, hypothermia, hepatitis, jaundice, ECG changes, photosensitivity, lowered seizure threshold, hematologic changes, hepatitis, rash.

For agent-specific side effects, see individual medication sections.

IX. Antipsychotic Interactions

1. Antacids and cimetidine - absorption of antipsychotics may be inhibited.
2. Anticholinergics, antihistamines, antiadrenergics - additive effects.
3. Antihypertensives - may potentiate hypotension (e.g., ACE Inhibitors); may inhibit neuronal uptake of clonidine and alpha-methyldopa.
4. Anticonvulsants - may increase metabolism and decrease level of antipsychotic; phenothiazines may decrease metabolism/ increase level of phenytoin.
5. Antidepressants - tricyclics and fluoxetine may reduce metabolism and increase levels of antipsychotics.
6. Antipsychotics - may increase levels of tricyclics.
7. Barbiturates - may increase metabolism and decrease levels of antipsychotics; may cause respiratory depression.
8. Cigarettes - may increase metabolism and decrease level of antipsychotics.
9. CNS depressants (including alcohol) - may cause CNS depression.
10. Digoxin - absorption may be increased.
11. Isoniazid - may cause hepatic toxicity, encephalopathy.
12. L-Dopa - effects blocked by dopamine antagonists.
13. Lithium - increases risk of neuroleptic-induced encephalopathic syndrome or neurotoxicity.
14. Oral contraceptives - may increase metabolism and decrease levels of antipsychotics.
15. Propranolol - levels of both agents may be increased.
16. Warfarin - highly protein-bound, may alter antipsychotic levels; levels may be decreased leading to decreased bleeding time.

For agent-specific interactions, see individual medication sections.

X. Preexisting Medical Conditions:

1. Cardiac history - use high potency agent (other than pimozide) to avoid conduction abnormalities.
2. Elderly - more sensitive to side effects; start with low dose of high potency

agent and increase slowly; bedtime doses reduce risk of problems with orthostatic hypotension, static hypotension.

3. Hematologic disorder - clozapine contraindicated.
4. Hepatic, renal, cardiac, respiratory disease - use antipsychotics with caution; monitor renal, cardiac, and liver function.
5. Parkinson's disease - anticholinergic effects of low potency agents may be beneficial.
6. Prostatic hypertrophy - agents with high anticholinergic activity are contraindicated.
7. Seizure history - some studies suggest that molindone may have lower seizure risk than other antipsychotics. Avoid loxapine and clozapine.
8. Pregnancy - phenothiazines may increase risk of anomalies. Avoid low potency agents.
9. Fluphenazine, haloperidol, trifluoperazine, and perphenazine are associated with lower risks during pregnancy.

X. **Managing Side Effects:**
   A. **Neuroleptic Malignant Syndrome** is an uncommon side effect with possible fatal outcome. Neuroleptic malignant syndrome is marked by elevated temperature, autonomic instability, delirium, and rigid muscle tone developing over 24-72 hrs. Risk factors for neuroleptic malignant syndrome include dehydration, heat exhaustion, and poor nutrition. Treatment includes:
      1. Discontinue antipsychotic.
      2. Monitor vital signs closely and transfer to an intensive care ward if autonomic instability develops.
      3. Check WBC, CPK, myoglobin, and liver enzymes.
      4. Cooling measures.
      5. Monitor renal output.
      6. Dantrolene (Dantrium): see medication listing.
      7. Bromocriptine (Parlodel): see medication listing.
   B. **Agranulocytosis** - most common with clozapine (1-2% incidence).
      1. Clozapine should be discontinued if WBC drops below 3,000/ mcl or 50% of the patient's normal level.
      2. Consider hematology consult.
   C. **Tardive Dyskinesia (TD)** is a neurological impairment, primarily limited to patients with history of chronic neuroleptic administration (greater than two months). TD may result in permanent dysfunction of facial (e.g., cheeks and lips), neck, or extremity motor function. Treatment may include:
      1. Monitor dyskinetic movements with abnormal involuntary movement scale which rates the degree of neurological

dysfunction.
2. Reduce or stop antipsychotic if possible.
3. If continued antipsychotic is necessary, consider change to an atypical agent.
4. Some studies suggest that vitamin E offers modest benefits in prevention and treatment of TD.

D. Dystonic reactions are characterized by painful, acute involuntary muscle spasms. They are common side effects of typical antipsychotic agents. Dystonic reactions commonly involve the patient's extremities. The muscle contractions are not life-threatening, unless they involve airway passages (e.g., larynx) and lead to shortness of breath. Treatment may include:
1. IM or IV antiparkinsonian agent:
   a. Benztropine (Cogentin) - 50 mg PO, IM, IV
   b. Or, Diphenhydramine (Benadryl) - 50 mg PO, IM, IV
2. Consider change of antipsychotic to relieve patient fears.
3. Prophylaxis against further episodes of dystonia with an oral anticholinergic agent such as benztropine (Cogentin), 2 mg PO bid for two weeks.
4. If dystonic reactions occur after discontinuing anticholinergic agent, longer prophylactic treatment should be provided (e.g., 3-6 months).

E. Drug-induced Parkinsonian Symptoms include bradykinesia, tremor, cogwheel rigidity, masked facies, and festinating gait. Treatments include:
1. Decreasing antipsychotic dose, if possible.
2. Short-moderate term use of anticholinergic (e.g., benztropine).
3. Consider changing to lower potency agent.

F. Akathisia is characterized by an intense sense of a need to move, manifesting as restlessness or anxiety. Treatments include:
1. Decreasing antipsychotic dose, if possible.
2. Trial of anticholinergic agent (e.g., benztropine 2 mg PO bid) if patient taking high potency agent.
3. Trial of beta-adrenergic antagonist such as propranolol, 10-30 mg PO tid.
4. Trial of a benzodiazepine such as clonazepam, 0.5 mg PO bid.
5. Consider changing to lower potency agent.

XI. Overdose
A. Death is uncommon with antipsychotic overdose. Risk of fatality is increased by concurrent use of alcohol or other CNS depressant.

B. Mesoridazine, pimozide, and thioridazine are associated with the greatest risk of fatality due to possible heart block and ventricular tachycardia.

C. CNS depression, hypotension, convulsions, fever, ECG changes, hypothermia, and hyperthermia are possible.

D. Treatment may include lavage, catharsis, IV diazepam treatment of seizure, and medical treatment of hypotension.

High Potency Antipsychotics

Haloperidol (Haldol)

Class: Butyrophenone
Mechanism: Dopamine-2 receptor antagonism
Indications: Psychotic disorders (e.g., schizophrenia), Tourette's Syndrome.
Preparations:
>Haloperidol tablets - 0.5, 1, 2, 5, 10, 20 mg
>Haloperidol lactate - 2 mg/ml conc.(PO), 5 mg/ml soln.(IM)
>Haloperidol decanoate - 50, 100 mg/ml (IM - depot)

Dosage:
>Moderate symptoms: 0.5-2.0 mg PO bid/tid
>Severe symptoms: Titrate to 3.0-5.0 mg PO bid/tid
>Maintenance: 5-20 PO mg/day
>Acute agitation: 2.0-5.0 IM q 30 min. prn
>Elderly: 0.5-20 mg PO bid/tid
>Chronic noncompliance: Switch to haloperidol decanoate at 10-15 times daily dose, given on monthly basis. Maximum single dose of 100 mg/day IM. Give balance of dose 4-5 days later if necessary.

Time to Onset: Sedation occurs in 15-30 minutes with IM dose. Resolution of psychosis occurs in days to months (usually 2-3 weeks).
Therapeutic Level: 5-20 ng/ml
Side Effect Profile: Orthostatic   hypotension (low), sedation(low), anticholinergic (low), extrapyramidal symptoms (high). Also, see antipsychotic side effect list.
Interactions: Fluoxetine may increase extrapyramidal symptoms of haloperidol. Also, see antipsychotic interaction list.
Major Safety Concerns: Neuroleptic malignant syndrome, tardive dyskinesia, dystonic reactions are possible (see general principles of antipsychotic use for details).
Augmentation: Concurrent use of benzodiazepines (e.g., 1-2 mg IM lorazepam) may reduce the amount of antipsychotic required for agitation control.
Advantages/ Disadvantages: High potency agents have less sedative, hypotensive, and anticholinergic side effects.   Many patients require concurrent use of antiparkinsonian agent (e.g., benztropine) to control extrapyramidal symptoms.

Pimozide (Orap)

Class: Diphenylbutylpiperdines
Mechanism: Dopamine-2 receptor antagonism
Indications: Tourette's Syndrome, psychotic disorders
Preparations: 2.0 mg tablets
Dosages:
  Tourette's: 0.5-1 mg bid, then increase dose every other day as needed (max. 0.2 mg/kg/day or 10 mg)
  Antipsychotic maintenance: 1-10 mg/day
Time to Onset: 2-4 hours to peak level, days-months (usually 2-3 weeks) for full antipsychotic effect.
Therapeutic Level: Not established
Contraindications: Pimozide is contraindicated in patients with a history of cardiac arrhythmia or with drugs that prolong QT interval.
Side Effect Profile: Orthostatic hypotension (low), sedation (low), anticholinergic (low), extrapyramidal symptoms (high). ECG changes include prolongation of QT interval. Also, see antipsychotic side effect list.
Interactions: Pimozide may alter effects of antiarrhythmic agents. Also, see antipsychotic interaction list.
Major Safety Concerns: Pimozide may cause ECG changes. Use caution in patients with a history of hypokalemia. Neuroleptic malignant syndrome, tardive dyskinesia, and dystonic reactions are possible (see general principles of antipsychotic use for details).
Augmentation: Concurrent use of benzodiazepines (e.g., 1-2 mg IM lorazepam) may reduce the amount of antipsychotic required for agitation control.
Advantages/Disadvantages: High potency agents have less sedative, hypotensive, and anticholinergic side effects. Many patients require concurrent use of antiparkinsonian agent (e.g.. benztropine) to control extrapyramidal symptoms. **Cardiac side effects** of pimozide make haloperidol safer first line treatment for Tourette's Syndrome.

Thiothixene (Navane)

Class: Thioxanthene
Mechanism: Dopamine-2 receptor antagonism
Indications: Psychotic disorders (e.g.. schizophrenia)
Preparations: Capsules - 1, 2, 5, 10, 20 mg
Thiothixene hydrochloride - 5 mg/ml conc.(PO); 5 mg/ml soln.(IM)
Dosage:
> Moderate symptoms: 2-5 mg PO/IM tid
> Severe symptoms: Titrate to 20-30 mg/day in divided doses (max. 60 mg/day)
> Acute agitation: 5 mg IM bid prn
> Maintenance: 5-30 mg/day

Time to Onset: Sedation occurs in 15-30 minutes with IM dose. Antipsychotic effect occurs in days-months (usually 2-3 weeks).
Therapeutic Level: Not established. Some suggest 2-57 ng/ml.
Side Effect Profile: Orthostatic hypotension (low), sedation (low), anticholinergic (low), extrapyramidal symptoms (high). Also, see antipsychotic side effect list.
Interactions: No thiothixene-specific interactions. See antipsychotic interaction list.
Major Safety Concerns: Neuroleptic malignant syndrome, tardive dyskinesia, and dystonic reactions are possible (see general principles of antipsychotic use for details).
Augmentation: Concurrent use of lorazepam ,1-2 mg IM, may lessen the antipsychotic dose requirement for agitation control.
Advantages/Disadvantages: High potency agents have low sedation, anticholinergic, and hypotensive side effects, but may require concurrent use of antiparkinsonian agent (e.g., benztropine) to control extrapyramidal symptoms.

Trifluoperazine (Stelazine)

Class: Piperazine
Mechanism: Dopamine-2 receptor antagonism
Indications: Psychotic disorders (e.g., schizophrenia)
Preparations: 1, 2, 5, 10 mg tabs; 10 mg/ml conc.(PO), 2 mg/ml soln. (IM)
Dosage:
> Moderate symptoms: 2-5 mg PO bid. Titrate to 15-20 mg/day.
> Severe symptoms: Titrate to 20-40 mg/day in divided doses

Acute agitation: 1-2 mg IM q4-6hrs. prn (max. of 6 mg/day). Do not
 repeat doses in less than 4 hrs.

Maintenance: 5-20 mg/day

Elderly: 1-15 mg/day

Time to Onset: Sedation occurs in 15-30 minutes with IM dose. Antipsychotic
effect occurs in days-months (usually 2-3 weeks).

Therapeutic Level: Not established

Side Effect Profile: Orthostatic hypotension (low), sedation (low),
anticholinergic (low), extrapyramidal symptoms (high). Also, see antipsychotic
side effect list.

Interactions: No trifluoperazine-specific interactions. See antipsychotic
interaction list.

Major Safety Concerns: Neuroleptic malignant syndrome, tardive dyskinesia,
and dystonic reactions are possible (see general principles of antipsychotic
use for details).

Augmentation: Concurrent use of lorazepam ,1-2 mg IM, may lessen the
antipsychotic dose requirement for agitation control.

Advantages/Disadvantages: High potency agents have low sedation,
anticholinergic, and hypotensive side effects, but may require concurrent use
of antiparkinsonian agent (e.g., benztropine) to control extrapyramidal
symptoms.

Mid-Potency Antipsychotics

Loxapine (Loxitane)

Class: Dibenzoxapine
Mechanism: Dopamine-2 receptor antagonism
Indications: Psychotic disorders (e.g., schizophrenia)
Preparations: 5, 10, 25, 50 mg; 25 mg/ml conc. (PO);
50 mg/ml soln. (IM)
Dosage:

> Moderate symptoms: 10 mg PO bid/tid. Titrate to 20-100 mg/day in
> divided doses, then change to qhs dosing.
> Severe symptoms: 10-20 mg bid/tid. Titrate as needed (max. 250
> mg/day).
> Acute agitation: 12.5-50 mg IM q4-6h. prn
> Maintenance: 50-100 mg/day
> Elderly: 5-250 mg/day

Time to Onset: Sedation occurs in 15-30 minutes with IM dose. Antipsychotic
effect occurs in days-months (usually 2-3 weeks).
Therapeutic Level: Not established
Side Effect Profile: Orthostatic hypotension (moderate), sedation
(moderate), anticholinergic (moderate), extrapyramidal symptoms (high). Also,
see antipsychotic side effect list.
Interactions: Avoid medications which lower the seizure threshold. Also, see
antipsychotic interaction list.
Major Safety Concerns: Neuroleptic malignant syndrome, tardive dyskinesia,
and dystonic reactions are possible (see general principles of antipsychotic
use for details).
Contraindications: Avoid medications which lower the seizure threshold.
Advantages/Disadvantages: Anticholinergic side effects of mid-potency
agents lessen the need for medication to control extrapyramidal side effects.
Loxapine may be associated with a higher **risk of seizure** than other high and
mid-potency agents.

Molindone (Moban)

Class: Dihydroindolones
Mechanism: Dopamine-2 receptor antagonism
Indications: Psychotic disorders (e.g., schizophrenia)
Preparations: 5, 10, 25, 100 mg tabs; 20 mg/ml conc. (PO)
Dosage:
> Moderate symptoms: 5-15 mg PO tid/qid
> Severe symptoms: Titrate to 10-40 mg tid/qid (max. 225 mg/day)
> Maintenance: 50-100 mg/day

Time to Onset: Peak sedation occurs in 2-3h. Antipsychotic effect occurs in days-months (usually 2-3 weeks).
Therapeutic Level: Not established
Side Effect Profile: Orthostatic hypotension (low), sedation (moderate), anticholinergic (moderate), extrapyramidal symptoms (high). Also, see antipsychotic side effect list.
Interactions: No molindone-specific interactions. See antipsychotic interaction list.
Major Safety Concerns: Neuroleptic malignant syndrome, tardive dyskinesia, and dystonic reactions are possible (see general principles of antipsychotic use for details).
Advantages/Disadvantages: Anticholinergic side effects of mid-potency agents lessen the need for medication to control extrapyramidal side effects. Studies suggest molindone is associated with **less weight gain**, amenorrhea, and impotence than other typical antipsychotics. Molindone appears less likely to cause seizures than other antipsychotics.

Perphenazine (Trilafon)

Class: Piperazine
Mechanism: Dopamine-2 receptor antagonism
Indications: Psychotic disorders (e.g., schizophrenia). Severe nausea and vomiting in adults.
Preparations: 2, 4, 8, 16 mg tabs; 16 mg/5 ml conc.(PO); 5 mg/ml soln.(IM)
Dosage:
> Moderate symptoms: 4-8 mg tid
> Severe symptoms: 8-16 mg bid/tid (max. 64 mg/day)
> Acute agitation: 5-10 mg IM q 6h. prn (max. 30 mg/day)
> Maintenance: 4-40 mg/day

Time to Onset: Sedation occurs in 15-30 minutes with IM dose. Antipsychotic effect occurs in days-months (usually 2-3 weeks).

Therapeutic Level: 0.8-2.4 ng/ml

Side Effect Profile: Orthostatic hypotension (low), sedation (low), anticholinergic (low), extrapyramidal symptoms (high). Also, see antipsychotic side effect list.

Interactions: No perphenazine-specific interactions. See antipsychotic interaction list.

Major Safety Concerns: Neuroleptic malignant syndrome, tardive dyskinesia, and dystonic reactions are possible (see general principles of antipsychotic use for details).

Advantages/Disadvantages: Anticholinergic side effects of mid-potency agents lessen the need for medication to control extrapyramidal side effects.

Prochlorperazine (Compazine)

Class: Piperazine

Mechanism: Dopamine-2 receptor antagonism

Indications: Psychotic disorders (e.g., schizophrenia) and, severe nausea and vomiting.

Preparations:

Prochlorperazine maleate: 5, 10, 25 mg tabs

Prochlorperazine maleate sustained release caps.: 10, 15 mg

Prochlorperazine suppository: 2.5, 5, 25 mg (PR)

Prochlorperazine edisylate: 5 mg/ml soln.(IM); 1 mg/ml conc.(PO)

Dosage:

> Moderate symptoms: 5-10 mg tid/qid
>
> Severe symptoms: 20-50 mg tid/qid
>
> Acute agitation: 10-20 mg IM q 2-4h. prn
>
> Maintenance: 50-150 mg/day

Time to Onset: Sedation occurs in 15-30 minutes with IM dose. Antipsychotic effect occurs in days-months (usually 2-3 weeks).

Therapeutic Level: Not established

Side Effect Profile: Orthostatic hypotension (low), sedation (moderate), anticholinergic (low), extrapyramidal symptoms (high). Also, see antipsychotic side effect list.

Interactions: No prochlorperazine-specific interactions. See antipsychotic interaction list.

Major Safety Concerns: Neuroleptic malignant syndrome, tardive dyskinesia, and dystonic reactions are possible (see general principles of antipsychotic use for details).

Advantages/Disadvantages: Anticholinergic side effects of mid-potency agents lessen the need for medication to control extrapyramidal side effects. Prochlorperazine is approved for IV use with severe nausea and vomiting (2.5-10 mg at less than 5 mg/min.).

Low Potency Antipsychotics

Chlorpromazine (Thorazine)

Class: Aliphatic Phenothiazine
Mechanism: Dopamine-2 receptor antagonism
Indications: Psychotic disorders (e.g., schizophrenia). Severe nausea and vomiting. Mania.
Preparations:
   Tablets: 10, 25, 50, 100, 200 mg
   Slow release capsules: 30, 75, 150 mg
   Oral liquid preparations: 30 mg/ml and 100 mg/ml conc.; 10 mg/5 ml syrup
   Injection solution: 25 mg/ml (IM)
   Suppositories: 25, 100 mg (PR)
Dosage:
   Moderate symptoms: 10-50 mg PO bid-qid (usually 400 mg/day)
   Severe symptoms: Titrate to 200-600 mg/day in divided doses (max. 2000 mg/day)
   Acute agitation: 25-50 mg IM q 4-6h. Increase slowly to maximum dose of 800 mg/day.
   Maintenance: 300-800 mg/day
   Elderly: 25-300 mg/day
Time to Onset: Sedation occurs in 15-30 minutes with IM dose. Antipsychotic effect occurs in days-months (usually 2-3 weeks).
Therapeutic Level: 30-100 mg/ml
Side Effect Profile: Orthostatic hypotension (high), sedation (high), anticholinergic (high), extrapyramidal symptoms (low). Also, see antipsychotic side effect list. Higher risk than most other typical antipsychotics for seizure, jaundice, photosensitivity, agranulocytosis, skin discoloration (bluish), granular deposits in lens and cornea. Prolongation of QT and PR intervals, blunting of T-waves, ST segment depression. Also, see antipsychotic side effect list.
Interactions: Strong potentiation of anticholinergics, antihistamines, antiadrenergics. Also, see antipsychotic interaction list.
Major Safety Concerns: Neuroleptic malignant syndrome, tardive dyskinesia, and dystonic reactions are possible (see general principles of antipsychotic use for details). Chlorpromazine has high lethality in overdose. It has a higher risk than many other antipsychotics for life-threatening agranulocytosis. Use chlorpromazine with caution in patients with a history of cardiovascular, liver,

or renal disease. Avoid use of chlorpromazine in pregnancy (especially in weeks 6-10).

Advantages/Disadvantages: Anticholinergic side effects of low potency agents lessen the need for medication to control extrapyramidal side effects. Chlorpromazine is the **most sedating antipsychotic**. It is associated with a high incidence of hypotensive and anticholinergic side effects.

Mesoridazine (Serentil)

Class: Piperidine
Mechanism: Dopamine-2 receptor antagonism
Indications: Psychotic disorders (e.g., schizophrenia)
Preparations: 10, 25, 50, 100 mg tablets; 25 mg/ml conc.(PO), 25 mg/ml (IM)
Dosage:
> Moderate symptoms: 25-50 mg po tid
> Severe symptoms: Titrate to 300 mg/day (max. 400 mg/day)
> Acute agitation: 25 mg IM. Dose may be repeated in 30 min. (max. 200 mg/day)
> Maintenance: 75-300 mg/day
> Elderly: 25-400 mg/day

Time to Onset: Sedation occurs in 15-30 minutes with IM dose. Antipsychotic effect occurs in days-months (usually 2-3 weeks).
Therapeutic Level: Not established
Side Effect Profile: Orthostatic hypotension (moderate), sedation (moderate), anticholinergic (high), extrapyramidal symptoms (moderate). Also, see antipsychotic side effect list.
Interactions: No mesoridazine-specific interactions. See antipsychotic interaction list.
Major Safety Concerns: Neuroleptic malignant syndrome, tardive dyskinesia, and dystonic reactions are possible (see general principles of antipsychotic use for details).
Advantages/Disadvantages: Anticholinergic side effects of low potency agents lessen the need for medication to control extrapyramidal side effects.

Thioridazine (Mellaril)

Class: Piperidine
Mechanism: Dopamine-2 receptor antagonism
Indications: Psychotic disorders (e.g., schizophrenia)
Preparations: 10, 15, 25, 50, 100, 200 mg tabs; 30 mg/ml and 100 mg/ml conc. (PO); 5 mg/ml susp. (PO)
Dosage:
>   Moderate symptoms: 25-100 mg tid
>   Severe symptoms: Titrate to 100-400 mg bid (max. 800 mg/day)
>   Acute agitation: No IM form available
>   Maintenance: 200-700 mg/day
>   Elderly: 10-300 mg/day

Time to Onset: Sedation occurs in 2-3 hrs. Antipsychotic effect occurs in days-months (usually 2-3 weeks).
Therapeutic Level: Not established
Side Effect Profile: Orthostatic hypotension (high), sedation (high), anticholinergic (high), extrapyramidal symptoms (low). Higher risk than most other antipsychotics for: **ECG** changes including marked T-wave changes, jaundice, decreased libido and retrograde ejaculation, and **pigmentation of retina**. Also, see antipsychotic side effect list.
Interactions: High potentiation of anticholinergic, antihistamine, antiadrenergic agents. See antipsychotic interaction list.
Major Safety Concerns: Neuroleptic malignant syndrome, tardive dyskinesia, and dystonic reactions are possible (see general principles of antipsychotic use for details). Permanent pigmentation of retina and potential blindness with doses above 800 mg/day is possible. Life-threatening agranulocytosis rarely occurs.
Advantages/Disadvantages: Thioridazine is very sedating. Anticholinergic side effects may reduce the incidence of extrapyramidal symptoms. Thioridazine is associated with risks of several serious side effects.

Atypical Antipsychotics

Clozapine (Clozaril)

Class: Dibenzodiazepine
Mechanism: Multiple receptor antagonism: serotonin-2, alpha-1&2 adrenergic, muscarinic-cholinergic, histamine-1, and dopamine-1.
Indications: Psychotic disorders (e.g., schizophrenia) which are refractory to treatment with typical antipsychotics. Also, psychotic patients with tardive dyskinesia or intolerable side effects.
Preparations: 25, 100 mg tabs
Dosage:
> Initially: 12.5 mg bid, then increase by 25 mg every 2-3 days to 100 mg tid
> Moderate symptoms: 300-400 mg/day in divided doses
> Severe symptoms: 400-600 mg/day (rare use up to 900 mg/day)
> Acute agitation: No IM dose available
> Maintenance: 400-600 mg/day

Time to Onset: Peak plasma level occurs in 1-4 hrs. Antipsychotic effect occurs in days-months (usually 1-6 weeks).
Therapeutic Level: > 350 ng/ml
Side Effect Profile: Orthostatic hypotension (high), sedation (high), anticholinergic (high), extrapyramidal symptoms (low).   Most common: sedation, dizziness, hypotension, tachycardia, constipation, hyperthermia, hypersalivation.   Shares many side effects with low potency typical antipsychotics but displays no EPS or prolactin changes.   Also, see antipsychotic list.
Interactions:
> **A.** Anticholinergic, antihistamine, and antiadrenergic - potentiation
> **B.** Cimetidine (Tagamet) - may increase clozapine levels. Use ranitidine (Zantac) instead.
> **C.** CNS depressants - potentiation
> **D.** Fluoxetine - may increase clozapine levels
> **E.** Lithium - may produce seizure, movement disorder, confusion
> **F.** TCAs - risk for seizure, cardiac changes, sedation
> **G.** Also, clozapine's list of interactions has considerable overlap with that of typical low potency agents (see antipsychotic interaction list).

Contraindications: Clozapine is contraindicated in patients with a history of hematologic disorders or epilepsy. Do not use clozapine with drugs which suppress bone marrow or have risk of agranulocytosis (e.g., carbamazepine, sulfonamides, captopril).

Major Safety Concerns:

1. Clozapine has a 1-2% incidence of **agranulocytosis.** Discontinue the drug if the WBC drops below 3,000/mcL or 50% of patient's normal count, or if granulocyte count drops below 1,500/mcL. Physicians should register with Clozaril National Registry (1-800-448-5938).

2. A 5% incidence of **seizure** has been noted in patients taking more than 600 mg/day of clozapine. The rate is 1-2% in patients taking less than 300 mg/day. If seizures develop, discontinue drug use and consider restarting with concurrent use of divalproex sodium (Depakote). Avoid use of drugs which lower the seizure threshold.

3. Use clozapine with caution and low doses in patients with hepatic or renal disease.

4. Monitor patients for hypotension and tachycardia (especially in first month).

Advantages/Disadvantages: Minimal to no risk of tardive dyskinesia. Rare cases of neuroleptic malignant syndrome. Clozapine is often effective against symptoms that are resistant to typical agents. It is more effective than typical agents in treatment of the negative symptoms of schizophrenia. Clozapine may be particularly useful in patients with Parkinson's disease and psychosis. It requires careful tapering to discontinue use. Major safety concerns are noted above. Clozapine use **requires weekly WBCs.**

Olanzapine (Zyprexa)

Class: Thiobenzodiazepine

Mechanism: Serotonin-2, dopamine-2 and, alpha-1 adrenergic antagonism.

Indications: Psychotic disorders (e.g., schizophrenia); final FDA approval is expected by January 1997.

Preparations: 5, 7.5, 10 mg tablets

Dosage:

> Initially: 5 mg/day, then gradually increase to 10-15 mg/day (10 mg is usually effective)
>
> Range: 5-20 mg/day

Time to Onset: Antipsychotic effect occurs in days-months.

Therapeutic Level: Not established.

Side Effect Profile: Orthostatic hypotension (moderate), sedation (high), anticholinergic (high), extrapyramidal symptoms (low). Most common side

effects: Insomnia, dry mouth, akathisia, nervousness, agitation. Also: Nausea, dyspepsia, tremor, light-headedness, orthostatic hypotension, and diaphoresis.
Interactions: Potentiation of antihistamine and anticholinergic agents. Olanzapine levels may be decreased by tobacco use and by carbamazepine due to enzyme induction. Olanzapine levels may be increased by fluvoxamine due to enzyme competition.
Major Safety Concerns: No tardive dyskinesia has been documented. Dystonic reactions are uncommon.
Advantages/Disadvantages: Olanzapine shares many of the advantages of clozapine but few of the safety risks. Olanzapine is more effective than typical agents in treatment of the negative symptoms of schizophrenia. Olanzapine is expected to be associated with a **very low incidence of tardive dyskinesia (TD)**. There is a **lower Incidence of extrapyramidal symptoms** with olanzapine than with risperidone.   There is no significant change in WBC with olanzapine. Its low seizure rate is comparable to the rate of typical agents.

Risperidone (Risperdal)

Class: Benzisoxazole
Mechanism: Serotonin-2, dopamine-2 and, alpha-2 adrenergic antagonism.
Indications: Psychotic disorders (e.g., schizophrenia)
Preparations: 1, 2, 3, 4 mg tabs; 1 mg/ml oral soln
Dosage:
> Moderate symptoms: Initially, 1 mg bid, then, increase by 1 mg/day to 2-4 mg bid
> Severe symptoms: Titrate to 4 mg bid, then to max. of 16 mg/day if necessary. Acute agitation: No IM dose available
> Maintenance: 2-4 mg bid
> Elderly: 2-4 mg/day

Time to Onset: Peak levels occur in two hours. Antipsychotic effect occurs in days-months (usually 1-6 weeks).
Therapeutic Level: Not firmly established. However, optimal dose window appears to be 4-8 mg/ day with bid dosing.
Side Effect Profile: Orthostatic hypotension (moderate), sedation (moderate), anticholinergic (low), extrapyramidal symptoms (low).   Incidence of extrapyramidal symptoms is very low with doses less than 6 mg/day. Most common side effects: anxiety, insomnia, sedation, orthostasis/ dizziness, nausea, constipation, rhinitis/nasal stuffiness, tachycardia, sexual dysfunction, rash. May prolong QT interval (not clinically significant effect in otherwise

healthy patient).

Interactions: No risperidone-specific interactions. Some overlap with mid-potency typical agents. See antipsychotic interaction list. Interactions related to dopamine antagonism, however, do not apply.

Major Safety Concerns: Tardive dyskinesia, extrapyramidal symptoms and, dystonic reactions are uncommon (see general principles of antipsychotic use for details). An increased risk of seizure in patients with hyponatremia has been noted.

Advantages/Disadvantages: Risperidone shares most of the advantages of clozapine but few of the safety risks. Risperidone is more effective than typical agents in treatment of the negative symptoms of schizophrenia. A low incidence of extrapyramidal symptoms is associated with doses less than 6 mg. Risperidone is associated with a **very low incidence of tardive dyskinesia (TD)**. At higher doses, it may actually reverse TD in some patients.

Anxiolytics and Hypnotics

Clinical Use of Anxiolytics and Hypnotics

I.   **Categories and Indications** - Anxiety and insomnia are primarily treated
with benzodiazepines and antidepressants.
   A.   **Benzodiazepines (Benzodiazepines)**, unlike barbiturates, have a
   high therapeutic index. The therapeutic dose is far below the dose
   for lethal overdose. Benzodiazepines also have the advantage of a
   lesser potential for abuse than barbiturates. Unlike the
   antidepressants, benzodiazepines have a rapid onset of anxiolytic
   effects. Long term use of benzodiazepines, however, is associated
   with tolerance and dependence problems.
   B.   **Antidepressants** are often effective in the long term treatment of
   anxiety and insomnia. Unlike benzodiazepines, the tricyclic
   antidepressants and serotonin-specific reuptake inhibitors are **not
   associated with tolerance or dependence**. SSRIs have the peculiar
   effect of decreasing anxiety in most patients but increases anxiety in
   others. Like the benzodiazepines, sedating antidepressants (e.g.,
   trazadone, doxepin) have a rapid onset of hypnotic effects.
   C.   **Barbiturates** have been almost completely replaced by the
   benzodiazepines. Several barbiturates, however, continue to be used
   within **very narrow ranges of treatment conditions** which are
   defined in the individual medication listings below.

II.   **Benzodiazepines**
   A.   **Side Effects**: Sedation, impaired concentration, ataxia, drowsiness,
   paradoxical agitation, vertigo, depression, memory impairment,
   confusion, GI complaints, hypotension, headache, disinhibition,
   dependence, withdrawal.
      1.   Short acting agents are associated with less unwanted sedation
      and are useful in treatment of early insomnia.
      2.   Long acting agents are associated with less withdrawal symptoms
      and are more useful in treatment of late insomnia..
      3.   Anterograde amnesia is more common with high potency agents.
   B.   **Benzodiazepine Interactions:**
      1.   CNS depressants such as alcohol, cyclic antidepressants and,
      anticonvulsants increase sedation and may lead to respiratory
      depression.

      2. Levodopa's antiparkinsonian effects may be reduced by benzodiazepines.

      3. Benzodiazepine levels may be increased by cimetidine, fluoxetine, ketoconazole, metoprolol, propranolol, estrogens, alcohol, erythromycin, disulfiram, valproic acid, and isoniazid.

      4. Benzodiazepine levels may be decreased by carbamazepine, rifampin, and antacids.

C. Preexisting Medical Problems

      1. Cognitive impairment may be exacerbated by benzodiazepines.

      2. COPD may be aggravated by benzodiazepines

      3. Benzodiazepines may be teratogenic or cause cardiac respiratory changes in newborns. Avoid benzodiazepines use in pregnancy and lactation. Patients should discontinue benzodiazepine use 1-2 months before planned conception.

      4. Sleep apnea may be exacerbated by benzodiazepines, leading to further impairment of respiration.

      5. Substance abuse history may predispose patients to benzodiazepine abuse and misuse.

      6. Use caution in patients with renal or hepatic disorders, porphyria, myasthenia gravis or, CNS depression.

D. Overdose is manifested by ataxia, hypotonia, nystagmus, coma. Treatment may include flumazenil (benzodiazepine receptor antagonist).

E. Withdrawal Symptoms may include anxiety, insomnia, irritability, fatigue, tremor, agitation, depression, abdominal discomfort, photosensitivity, psychosis and, seizure.

III. Barbiturates

A. Barbiturate Side Effects: CNS depression, nausea, vomiting, diarrhea, cramping, dependence, withdrawal (taper gradually), nightmares, paradoxical agitation, confusion, impaired coordination, rash, **high abuse potential.**

B. Barbiturate Interactions

      1. Barbiturates enhance the hepatic metabolism of narcotics, anticonvulsants, anticoagulants, antiarrhythmics, antidepressants, corticosteroids, estrogen and, progesterone.

      2. CNS depressants such as alcohol, cyclic antidepressants and, antipsychotics will potentiate the CNS and respiratory depressant effects of barbiturates.

C. Preexisting Medical Problems

      1. Barbiturates are contraindicated in patients with a history of acute intermittent porphyria.

   2. Depression may exacerbated by barbiturates.
   3. Hepatic disease may be aggravated by barbiturates.
   4. Substance abuse history may be a contraindication for barbiturate use due to the high potential for drug misuse and abuse.
   5. Use caution in patients with diabetes, renal disorder, hyperthyroidism, hypoadrenalism or, anemia.
   6. Barbiturates should not be used in pregnancy due to potential teratogenic effects.
D. **Overdose** may be manifested by confusion, irritability, hyporeflexia, nystagmus, CNS depression and, coma.
E. **Withdrawal symptoms** are similar to those of benzodiazepines (noted above).

Benzodiazepines and Zolpidem

Alprazolam (Xanax)

Category: Benzodiazepine receptor agonist
Mechanism: Facilitates GABA attachment to GABA receptor
Indications: Anxiety disorders
Preparations: 0.025, 0.5, 1, 2 mg tabs
Dosage:
    Anxiety: 0.25-1.0 mg tid
    Panic disorder: 0.5-3 mg tid (max. 10 mg/day)
    Range of dosing: 0.5-10 mg/day
    Elderly: 0.5-6 mg/day
Half Life: 12 hrs.
Therapeutic Level: Not established. Some suggest 20-40 ng/ml.
Pharmacokinetics: Onset (fast), duration (short)
Side Effects: Sedation most common. See benzodiazepine side effect list.
Interactions: See benzodiazepine interaction list.
Major Safety Concerns: Warn patients about potentially hazardous activities such as driving. Use caution in patients with a history of acute intermittent porphyria. Advise potential childbearing patients of possibility of teratogenic effects (based on animal studies). Remain alert to the risks for dependence, withdrawal and, seizure.
Contraindications: Benzodiazepine use is contraindicated in patients with acute narrow angle glaucoma. Use is permitted with open angle glaucoma under treatment.
Advantages/Disadvantages: Fast onset provides quick relief of acute anxiety. Short duration of action is associated with **less unwanted sedation** than other benzodiazepines. High potency of alprazolam results in a greater incidence of cognitive deficits. Dependence is common with alprazolam. Abrupt discontinuation may result in intense withdrawal symptoms.

Chlordiazepoxide (Librium, Libritabs)

Category: Benzodiazepine receptor agonist
Mechanism: Facilitates GABA attachment to GABA receptor
Indications: Anxiety disorders and alcohol withdrawal
Preparations: 5, 10, 25 mg caps
100 mg powder + diluent for injection
Chlordiazepoxide (Libritabs) - 5, 25 mg tabs
Dosage:

> Anxiety: 5-25 mg PO tid/qid
> Alcohol withdrawal: 25-50 mg PO/IM every 2-4 hrs. prn signs of alcohol withdrawal (max. 100 mg/day) for 2-4 days.
> Long half life results in slow taper of blood level after fourth day. Lower doses are indicated if significant hepatic disorder is apparent (e.g., bilirubin elevation).
> Dose range: 10-100 mg/day
> Elderly: 5-100 mg/day

Half Life: 80-100 hrs.
Therapeutic Level: Not established
Pharmacokinetics: Onset (moderate), duration (long)
Side Effects: Sedation is most common. See benzodiazepine side effect list.
Interactions: See benzodiazepine interaction list.
Major Safety Concerns: Warn patients about potentially hazardous activities such as driving. Use caution in patients with a history of acute intermittent porphyria. Advise potential childbearing patients of possibility of teratogenic effects (based on animal studies). Remain alert to the risks for dependence, withdrawal and, seizure.
Contraindications: Benzodiazepine use is contraindicated in patients with acute narrow angle glaucoma. Use is permitted with open angle glaucoma under treatment.
Advantages/Disadvantages: Long duration of action may permit single daily dosing for anxiety. Chlordiazepoxide has a slower onset than Valium. Be careful not to quickly overload the patient in treatment of alcohol withdrawal.

Clonazepam (Klonopin)

Category: Benzodiazepine receptor agonist
Mechanism: Facilitates GABA attachment to GABA receptor
Indications: Approved as anticonvulsant. Used widely as an anxiolytic and **mood stabilizer**.
Preparations: 0.5, 1, 2 mg tabs
Dosage:
    Anxiety: 0.25-6 mg/day (divided doses)
    Mood stabilization: 0.25-10 mg/day
    Dose range: 0.25-10 mg/day
    Elderly: 0.25-1.5 mg/day
Half Life: 20-50 hrs.
Therapeutic Level: Not established
Pharmacokinetics: Onset (fast), duration (long)
Side Effects: Sedation is most common. See benzodiazepine side effect list.
Interactions: See benzodiazepine interaction list.
Major Safety Concerns: Warn patients about potentially hazardous activities such as driving. Use caution in patients with a history of acute intermittent porphyria. Advise potential childbearing patients of possibility of teratogenic effects (based on animal studies). Remain alert to the risks for dependence, withdrawal and, seizure.
Contraindications: Benzodiazepine use is contraindicated in patients with acute narrow angle glaucoma. Use is permitted with open angle glaucoma under treatment.
Advantages/Disadvantages: Clonazepam has a wide range of uses. Its rapid onset provides prompt relief. Its long duration lessens withdrawal effects. Clonazepam may be substituted for shorter acting benzodiazepines, such as alprazolam, in the treatment of benzodiazepine dependence. Clonazepam does not provide the rapid euphoria sometimes noted with alprazolam. High potency agents such as clonazepam, however, have an increased incidence of cognitive side effects.

Clorazepate (Tranxene)

Category: Benzodiazepine receptor agonist
Mechanism: Facilitates GABA attachment to GABA receptor
Indications: Anxiety disorders and alcohol withdrawal
Preparations: 3.75, 7.5, 11.25, 15, 22.5 tabs; 3.75, 7.5, 15 mg caps
Dosage:

Anxiety: 7.5 mg PO tid or 15 qhs. Increase as needed.

Alcohol withdrawal: 7.5-15 mg q 2-4 hrs. prn signs of alcohol withdrawal (max. 90 mg/day) for 2-4 days. Long half life results in slow taper of blood levels after fourth day. Lower dose, if significant hepatic disorder is present (e.g., bilirubin elevation).

Dose range: 15-60 mg/day (max. 90 mg/day)

Elderly: 7.5-15 mg/day

Half Life: 100 hrs.

Therapeutic Level: Not established. Some suggest 600-1500 ng/ml of desmethyldiazepam metabolite.
Pharmacokinetics: Onset (fast), duration (long)
Side Effects: Sedation is most common. See benzodiazepine side effect list.
Interactions: See benzodiazepine interaction list.
Major Safety Concerns: Warn patients about potentially hazardous activities such as driving. Use caution in patients with a history of acute intermittent porphyria. Advise potential childbearing patients of possibility of teratogenic effects (based on animal studies). Remain alert to the risks for dependence, withdrawal and, seizure.
Contraindications: Benzodiazepine use is contraindicated in patients with acute narrow angle glaucoma. Use is permitted with open angle glaucoma under treatment.
Advantages/Disadvantages: Clorazepate has a faster onset than chlordiazepoxide in treatment of alcohol withdrawal. Its long duration of action permits once daily dosing for treatment of anxiety.

Diazepam (Valium)

Category: Benzodiazepine receptor agonist
Mechanism: Facilitates GABA attachment to GABA receptor
Indications: Anxiety disorders, alcohol withdrawal, adjunct treatment of muscle spasm and movement disorders.
Preparations: 2, 5, 10 mg tabs; 15 mg caps (sustained release); 5 mg/ml solution for IM, IV use
Dosage:

> Anxiety: 2-40 mg/day (divided doses)
>
> Alcohol withdrawal: 5-10 mg PO q 1-4 hrs. prn withdrawal signs for 2-4 days; or 5-10 mg IM/IV to initiate treatment or for resistant patient. Maximum of 60 mg/day (may be higher for severe dependance). Lower doses if significant hepatic disorder (e.g., bilirubin elevation).
>
> Dose range: 2-60 mg/day
>
> Elderly: 2.5-60 mg/day

Half Life: 100 hrs.
Therapeutic Level: Not established. Some suggest 300-100 ng/ml (same level for desmethyldiazepam).
Pharmacokinetics: Onset (fast), duration (long)
Side Effects: Sedation is most common. See benzodiazepine side effect list.
Interactions: See benzodiazepine interaction list.
Major Safety Concerns: Warn patients about potentially hazardous activities such as driving. Use caution in patients with a history of acute intermittent porphyria. Advise potential childbearing patients of possibility of teratogenic effects (based on animal studies). Remain alert to the risks for dependence, withdrawal and, seizure.
Contraindications: Benzodiazepine use is contraindicated in patients with acute narrow angle glaucoma. Use is permitted with open angle glaucoma under treatment.
Advantages/Disadvantages: Diazepam is the **most rapidly absorbed benzodiazepine**. It provides rapid control of **alcohol withdrawal** with oral dose. The long half life of diazepam results in a slow taper of blood levels after discontinuing use at day 3-4 of alcohol withdrawal treatment. A parenteral form is available.

Estazolam (ProSom)

Category: Benzodiazepine receptor agonist
Mechanism: Facilitates GABA attachment to GABA receptor
Indications: Insomnia
Preparations: 1, 2 mg tabs
Dosage:
   Insomnia: 1-2 mg qhs
   Elderly: 0.5-1.0 mg qhs
Half Life: 10-24 hrs.
Therapeutic Level: Not established
Pharmacokinetics: Onset (fast), duration (moderate)
Side Effects: See benzodiazepine side effect list.
Interactions: See benzodiazepine interaction list.
Major Safety Concerns: Warn patients about potentially hazardous activities such as driving. Use caution in patients with a history of acute intermittent porphyria. Advise potential childbearing patients of possibility of teratogenic effects (based on animal studies). Remain alert to the risks for dependence, withdrawal and, seizure.
Contraindications: Benzodiazepine use is contraindicated in patients with acute narrow angle glaucoma. Use is permitted with open angle glaucoma under treatment.
Advantages/Disadvantages: Fast onset of estazolam is useful for treatment of early insomnia. As a high potency agent, estazolam may have a higher incidence of cognitive side effects.

Flurazepam (Dalmane)

Category: Benzodiazepine receptor agonist
Mechanism: Facilitates GABA attachment to GABA receptor
Indications: Insomnia
Preparations: 15, 30 mg tabs
Dosage: Insomnia: 15-30 mg qhs (same for elderly)
Half Life: 100 hrs.
Therapeutic Level: Not established
Pharmacokinetics: Onset (fast), duration (long)
Side Effects: See benzodiazepine side effect list.
Interactions: See benzodiazepine interaction list.
Major Safety Concerns: Warn patients about potentially hazardous activities

such as driving. Use caution in patients with a history of acute intermittent porphyria. Advise potential childbearing patients of possibility of teratogenic effects (based on animal studies). Remain alert to the risks for dependence, withdrawal and, seizure.

Contraindications: Benzodiazepine use is contraindicated in patients with acute narrow angle glaucoma. Use is permitted with open angle glaucoma under treatment.

Advantages/Disadvantages: Fast onset is useful in treatment of early insomnia. Long duration is useful in treatment of late insomnia, but may result in morning sedation if taken late in evening.

Halazepam (Paxipam)

Category: Benzodiazepine receptor agonist (benzodiazepine-1 and benzodiazepine-2)

Mechanism: Facilitates GABA attachment to GABA receptor

Indications: Anxiety disorders

Preparations: 20, 40 mg tabs

Dosage:

    Anxiety: 20--80 mg/day (divided doses)

    Dose range: 40-160 mg/day

    Elderly: 20-160 mg/day

Half Life: 100 hrs.

Therapeutic Level: Not established

Pharmacokinetics: Onset (moderate), duration (long)

Side Effects: Sedation is most common. See benzodiazepine side effect list.

Interactions: See benzodiazepine interaction list.

Major Safety Concerns: Warn patients about potentially hazardous activities such as driving. Use caution in patients with a history of acute intermittent porphyria. Advise potential childbearing patients of possibility of teratogenic effects (based on animal studies). Remain alert to the risks for dependence, withdrawal and, seizure.

Contraindications: Benzodiazepine use is contraindicated in patients with acute narrow angle glaucoma. Use is permitted with open angle glaucoma under treatment.

Advantages/Disadvantages: Long half life of halazepam permits daily dosing and lessens withdrawal effects.

Lorazepam (Ativan)

Category: Benzodiazepine receptor agonist
Mechanism: Facilitates GABA attachment to GABA receptor
Indications: Anxiety disorders and insomnia. Also used for alcohol withdrawal if significant hepatic disorder present.
Preparations: 0.5, 1, 2 mg tabs; 2 mg/ml, 4 mg/ml soln. (IV, IM)
Dosage:

Anxiety: 0.5-6 mg/day (divided doses)

Alcohol withdrawal: 0.5-2 mg q 1-4 hrs. prn signs of alcohol withdrawal; or 0.5-1.0 mg IM to initiate treatment.

Maximum dose of 6 mg/day (may be higher for severe dependance). Lower doses if significant hepatic disorder is apparent (e.g., bilirubin elevation).

Insomnia: 0.5-2.0 mg qhs

Dose range: 1-6 mg/day

Elderly: 1-4 mg/day

Half Life: 12-15 hrs.
Therapeutic Level: Not established. Some suggest 20-80 ng/ml.
Pharmacokinetics: Onset (fast), duration (short)
Side Effects: Sedation is most common. See benzodiazepine side effect list.
Interactions: See benzodiazepine interaction list.
Major Safety Concerns: Warn patients about potentially hazardous activities such as driving. Use caution in patients with a history of acute intermittent porphyria. Advise potential childbearing patients of possibility of teratogenic effects (based on animal studies). Remain alert to the risks for dependence, withdrawal and, seizure.
Contraindications: Benzodiazepine use is contraindicated in patients with acute narrow angle glaucoma. Use is permitted with open angle glaucoma under treatment.
Advantages/Disadvantages: Short half life lorazepam permits use in the presence of significant **hepatic disorder**. Useful in alcohol withdrawal. Dosing interval should be increased based on amount of hepatic damage and level of sedation. Parenteral form is useful in **rapid control of agitation** resulting from variety of conditions (e.g., psychosis, drug-induced agitation). Short duration results in minimal AM sedation when used for insomnia. As a high potency agent, it may have a higher incidence of cognitive side effects.

Oxazepam (Serax)

Category: Benzodiazepine receptor agonist

Mechanism: Facilitates GABA attachment to GABA receptor

Indications: Anxiety disorders and alcohol withdrawal

Preparations: 10, 15, 30 mg caps; 15 mg tabs

Dosage:

    Anxiety: 30-120 mg/day (requires tid/qid dosing)

    Alcohol withdrawal: 15-30 mg q 2-4 hrs. prn signs of alcohol withdrawal. Maximum dose of 120 mg/day (may be higher for severe dependance). Lower doses if significant hepatic disorder is apparent (e.g., bilirubin elevation).

    Elderly - 30-100 mg/day

Half Life: 8 hrs.

Therapeutic Level: Not established

Pharmacokinetics: Onset (slow), duration (short)

Side Effects: Sedation is most common. See benzodiazepine side effect list.

Interactions: See benzodiazepine interaction list.

Major Safety Concerns: Warn patients about potentially hazardous activities such as driving. Use caution in patients with a history of acute intermittent porphyria. Advise potential childbearing patients of possibility of teratogenic effects (based on animal studies). Remain alert to the risks for dependence, withdrawal and, seizure.

Contraindications: Benzodiazepine use is contraindicated in patients with acute narrow angle glaucoma. Use is permitted with open angle glaucoma under treatment.

Advantages/Disadvantages: Short half life of oxazepam may be beneficial to patients with hepatic disorders. Slow absorption and short duration presents difficulty for titration treatment of alcohol withdrawal. Oxazepam requires tid/qid dosing.

Prazepam (Centrax)

Category: Benzodiazepine receptor agonist
Mechanism: Facilitates GABA attachment to GABA receptor
Indications: Anxiety disorders
Preparations: 5, 10, 20 mg caps; 10 mg tabs
Dosage:
  Anxiety: 20-60 mg day (divided doses or qhs)
  Elderly: 10-50 mg/day
Half Life: 100 hrs.
Therapeutic Level: Not established
Pharmacokinetics: Onset (slow), duration (long)
Side Effects: Sedation is most common. See benzodiazepine side effect list.
Interactions: Benzodiazepine interaction list.
Major Safety Concerns: Warn patients about potentially hazardous activities such as driving. Use caution in patients with a history of acute intermittent porphyria. Advise potential childbearing patients of possibility of teratogenic effects (based on animal studies). Remain alert to the risks for dependence, withdrawal and, seizure.
Contraindications: Benzodiazepine use is contraindicated in patients with acute narrow angle glaucoma. Use is permitted with open angle glaucoma under treatment.
Advantages/Disadvantages: Long duration of action may lead to unwanted sedation.

Quazepam (Doral)

Category: Benzodiazepine receptor agonist
Mechanism: Facilitates GABA attachment to GABA receptor
Indications: Insomnia
Preparations: 7.5, 15 mg tabs
Dosage:
  Insomnia: 7.5-15 mg qhs
  Dose range: 7.5-30 mg qhs
  Elderly: 7.5 mg qhs
Half Life: 100 hrs.
Therapeutic Level: Not established
Pharmacokinetics: Onset (fast), duration (long)
Side Effects: See benzodiazepine side effect list.

Interactions: See benzodiazepine interaction list.

Major Safety Concerns: Warn patients about potentially hazardous activities such as driving. Use caution in patients with a history of acute intermittent porphyria. Advise potential childbearing patients of possibility of teratogenic effects (based on animal studies). Remain alert to the risks for dependence, withdrawal and, seizure.

Contraindications: Benzodiazepine use is contraindicated in patients with acute narrow angle glaucoma. Use is permitted with open angle glaucoma under treatment.

Advantages/Disadvantages: Long duration of quazepam may result in morning sedation with late evening use.

Temazepam (Restoril)

Category: Benzodiazepine receptor agonist

Mechanism: Facilitates GABA attachment to GABA receptor

Indication: Insomnia

Preparations: 7.5, 15, 30 mg caps

Dosage: Insomnia: 7.5-30 mg qhs (same for elderly)

Half Life: 10-12 hrs.

Therapeutic Level: Not established

Pharmacokinetics: Onset (moderate), duration (short)

Side Effects: See benzodiazepine side effect list.

Interactions: See benzodiazepine interaction list.

Major Safety Concerns: Warn patients about potentially hazardous activities such as driving. Use caution in patients with a history of acute intermittent porphyria. Advise potential childbearing patients of possibility of teratogenic effects (based on animal studies). Remain alert to the risks for dependence, withdrawal and, seizure.

Contraindications: Benzodiazepine use is contraindicated in patients with acute narrow angle glaucoma. Use is permitted with open angle glaucoma under treatment.

Advantages/Disadvantages: Short duration of action limits morning sedation.

Triazolam (Halcion)

Category: Benzodiazepine receptor agonist
Mechanism: Facilitates GABA attachment to GABA receptor
Indication: Insomnia
Preparations: 0.125, 0.25 mg tabs
Dosage: Insomnia: 0.125-0.25 mg qhs (same for elderly)
Half Life: 2 hrs.
Therapeutic Level: Not established
Pharmacokinetics: Onset (fast), duration (short)
Side Effects: See benzodiazepine side effect list.
Interactions: See benzodiazepine interaction list.
Major Safety Concerns: Warn patients about potentially hazardous activities such as driving. Use caution in patients with a history of acute intermittent porphyria. Advise potential childbearing patients of possibility of teratogenic effects (based on animal studies). Remain alert to the risks for dependence, withdrawal and, seizure.
Contraindications: Benzodiazepine use is contraindicated in patients with acute narrow angle glaucoma. Use is permitted with open angle glaucoma under treatment.
Advantages/Disadvantages: Ultra-short half life results in minimal AM sedation. High potency agents are associated with increased incidence of cognitive side effects. Recommended triazolam use is limited to 10 days.

Zolpidem (Ambien)

Category: Hypnotic
Mechanism: Binds to the benzodiazepine receptor complex, but zolpidem is not a benzodiazepine.
Indications: Insomnia
Preparations: 5, 10 mg tabs
Dosage:
    Insomnia: Approved at 10 mg qhs
    Occasionally used up to 15-20 mg qhs
    Elderly: 5 mg initial dose
Half Life: 2-3 hrs.
Pharmacokinetics: Onset (fast), duration (short)
Side Effects: Sedation, dizziness, GI upset, nausea, vomiting, anterograde amnesia, tolerance, dependence, abuse.
Interactions: Potentiation of other CNS depressants (e.g., alcohol).

Major Safety Concerns: Warn patients about potentially hazardous activities such as driving. Decrease the dose in patients with hepatic or renal impairment. Zolpidem is not recommended for long term use.

Advantages/Disadvantages: Zolpidem has a rapid onset. It is useful for inhibiting and maintaining sleep. Zolpidem use results in less tolerance and withdrawal effects than other benzodiazepines. It lacks the muscle relaxation effects of the benzodiazepines. Time of recommended use is limited to 7-10 days. Zolpidem is much more expensive than benzodiazepine hypnotics.

Barbiturates

Amobarbital (Amytal)

Category: Sedative-hypnotic

Mechanism: Binds to benzodiazepine-GABA receptor complex and enhances GABA activity.

Indications: Current use is limited to differential diagnosis of some somatoform disorders and catatonia.

Preparations: 30, 50, 100 mg tabs; 65, 200 mg caps; 250 mg/5 ml, 500 mg/5 ml solution (IM, IV)

Dosage:
    Sedation: 50-100 mg
    Hypnosis: 50-200 mg (max. 400 mg/day)

Half Life: 8-42 hrs.

Side Effects: CNS depression, nausea, impaired motor coordination. Also, see barbiturate side effect list.

Interactions: Enhances hepatic metabolism of other agents. Also, see barbiturate interaction list.

Major Safety Concerns: Barbiturates have high abuse potential and lethality in overdose (respiratory depression). They potentiate CNS depression of other agents, including alcohol. Also, see cautions for preexisting medical conditions in general principles of barbiturate use.

Contraindications: Do not use barbiturates in patients with a history of acute intermittent porphyria. Avoid barbiturate use in pregnancy (potential teratogenic effects).

Advantages/Disadvantages: Barbiturates have higher **abuse potential and lethality** in overdose than benzodiazepines. Lorazepam is equally effective for inducing hypnotic states and carries lower risk of respiratory depression.

Methohexital (Brevital)

Category: General anesthetic

Mechanism: Binds to BB-GABA receptor complex and enhances GABA activity.

Indications: Psychiatric use is limited to anesthesia for electroconvulsive therapy (ECT).

Preparations: 500 mg/ 50 ml solution (IV)

Dosage:

> Anesthesia: Individualized dosing; approximately 6.75 mg/kg for initial ECT treatment.

Half Life: 3-6 hrs.

Side Effects: CNS depression, nausea, impaired motor coordination. See barbiturate side effect list.

Interactions: Enhances hepatic metabolism of other agents. See barbiturate interaction list.

Major Safety Concerns: Barbiturates have high abuse potential and lethality in overdose (respiratory depression). They potentiate CNS depression of other agents, including alcohol. Also, see cautions for preexisting medical conditions in general principles of barbiturate use.

Contraindications: Do not use barbiturates in patients with a history of acute intermittent porphyria. Avoid barbiturate use in pregnancy (potential teratogenic effects).

Advantages/Disadvantages: Barbiturates have higher **abuse potential and lethality** in overdose than benzodiazepines. Methohexital is associated with less risk of cardiac arrhythmia than other barbiturates. Methohexital's short half life is particularly useful for the brief time period required for electroconvulsive therapy.

Pentobarbital (Nembutal)

Category: Sedative-hypnotic

Mechanism: Binds to benzodiazepine-GABA receptor complex and enhances GABA activity.

Indications: Psychiatric use is limited to assessment and detoxification of CNS depressant (i.e., barbiturate) dependance.

Preparations: 50, 100 mg caps, 20 mg/ml conc (PO); 50 mg/ml soln. (IV, IM)

Dosage:

> Challenge dose: 200 mg PO. Repeat at 300 mg if no effect.
> Withdrawal dose: Dependent on level of dependence (tables available

elsewhere). Maximum dose of 600 mg/day. Decrease dose by 1/10 th each day (q 8 hr. dosing).

Half Life: 15-48 hrs.

Side Effects: CNS depression, nausea, impaired motor coordination. See barbiturate side effect list.

Interactions: Enhances hepatic metabolism of other agents. See barbiturate interaction list.

Major Safety Concerns: Barbiturates have high abuse potential and lethality in overdose (respiratory depression). They potentiate CNS depression of other agents, including alcohol. Also, see cautions for preexisting medical conditions in general principles of barbiturate use.

Contraindications: Do not use barbiturates in patients with a history of acute intermittent porphyria. Avoid barbiturate use in pregnancy (potential teratogenic effects).

Advantages/Disadvantages: Barbiturates have higher **abuse potential and lethality** in overdose than benzodiazepines. Pentobarbital may be used for both assessment and treatment barbiturate dependence.

Phenobarbital (Luminal)

Category: Sedative-Hypnotic

Mechanism: Binds to benzodiazepine-GABA receptor complex and enhances GABA activity.

Indications: Psychiatric use is limited to treatment of withdrawal from barbiturate dependence.

Preparations: 15, 30, 60, 100 mg tabs; 20 mg/5 ml elixir (PO); 130 mg/ml soln. (IV, IM)

Dosage:

Barbiturate withdrawal treatment: Dosage depends on level of dependance as determined by pentobarbital challenge. Maximum dose of 200 mg/day (tables available elsewhere).

Half Life: 80-130 hrs.

Side Effects: CNS depression, nausea, impaired motor coordination. See barbiturate side effect list.

Interactions: Enhances hepatic metabolism of other agents. See barbiturate interaction list.

Major Safety Concerns: Barbiturates have high abuse potential and lethality in overdose (respiratory depression). They potentiate CNS depression of other agents, including alcohol. Also, see cautions for preexisting medical conditions in general principles of barbiturate use.

Contraindications: Do not use barbiturates in patients with a history of acute intermittent porphyria. Avoid barbiturate use in pregnancy (potential teratogenic effects).

Advantages/Disadvantages: Barbiturates have higher **abuse potential and lethality** in overdose than benzodiazepines. Phenobarbital's long half life results in lower dosage requirements than pentobarbital in treatment of barbiturate withdrawal.

Other Anxiolytics and Hypnotics

Buspirone (BuSpar)

Category: Non-benzodiazepine anxiolytic
Mechanism: Serotonin 1A agonist
Indications: Anxiety disorders (e.g., generalized anxiety disorder). Also, used to augment antidepressant treatment of depression.
Preparations: 5, 10 mg tabs
Dosage:
> Initially: 5 mg tid, then increase by 5 mg every 3 days
> Dose range: 15-30 mg/day (max. 60 mg/day). Same dose range for elderly. Same dose range for antidepressant augmentation.

Half Life: 2-11 hrs.
Pharmacokinetics: Onset (moderate), duration (short)
Side Effects: Headache, nervousness, fatigue, dry mouth, GI distress, dizziness.
Interactions:
Fluoxetine may decrease effects of buspirone. Haloperidol may increase buspirone level. MAO-I may increase blood pressure.
Major Safety Concerns: Use caution in patients with renal or hepatic disease.
Contraindications: MAO-I use is contraindicated for two weeks before or after buspirone.
Advantages/Disadvantages: Buspirone lacks the sedation and dependence associated with benzodiazepines. It causes less cognitive impairment than benzodiazepines but is also less effective, especially in patients with prior experience with benzodiazepines. Buspirone may be used to augment fluoxetine treatment of depression or OCD. Buspirone is not useful for treating panic disorder. Its short half life requires tid dosing. Buspirone has a delayed onset of therapeutic effect (2-4 weeks).

Chloral Hydrate (Noctec)

Category: Hypnotic
Mechanism: CNS depression, specific mechanism is unknown
Indications: Past use in insomnia (especially with elderly). Current use is almost exclusively limited to sedation of children requiring surgical or diagnostic procedures.
Preparations: 250, 500 mg caps; 250 mg/5 ml and 500 mg/5 ml syrup (PO); 325, 500 mg supp. (PR).
Dosage:

>Adult insomnia: 500-100 mg qhs (short term only)
>Child sedation: See specialty text (some sources recommend 80-100 mg/kg; max. 3 grams).

Half Life: 8 hrs.
Pharmacokinetics: Onset (fast), duration (moderate)
Side Effects: Sedation, nausea, vomiting, diarrhea, impaired coordination, nightmares, paranoia, tolerance, dependance.
Interactions: Lasix, anticoagulants. Other CNS depressants.
Major Safety Concerns: Chloral hydrate is highly lethal in overdose. Dependance and withdrawal may be severe. Avoid use of chloral hydrate in patients with a history of porphyria.
Contraindications: Chloral hydrate is contraindicated in patients with gastritis, duodenal or gastric ulcers, hepatic, cardiac or hepatic disease.
Advantages/Disadvantages: Benzodiazepines are equally effective and have much safer side effect profile than chloral hydrate.

Diphenhydramine (Benadryl)

Category: Antihistamine, **antiparkinsonian agent**, hypnotic
Mechanism: Histamine receptor antagonist (sedation), acetylcholine receptor antagonist (extrapyramidal symptom control).
Indications: Insomnia (brief treatment), neuroleptic-induced extrapyramidal symptoms (EPS).
Preparations: 25, 50 mg tabs; 25, 50 mg caps; 50 mg/ml soln. (IM, IV); 12.5 mg/5 ml elixir (PO)
Dosage:

>Insomnia: 50 mg PO qhs (100 mg dose is not more effective)
>Antiparkinson's: 25-50 mg PO q6-8 hrs.
>Acute EPS: 25-50 mg IV, IM

Half Life: 1-4 hrs.

Pharmacokinetics: Onset (moderate), duration (short)

Side Effects: Dry mouth, dizziness, drowsiness, tremor, thickening of bronchial secretions, hypotension, decreased motor coordination, GI distress.

Interactions: Anticholinergics, MAO-I, Demerol, CNS depressants. Increases level of phenytoin.

Major Safety Concerns: Warn patients about potentially hazardous activities such as driving. Use caution in patients with a history of urine retention, asthma, open angle glaucoma, peptic ulcer disease, hyperthyroidism, hepatic or, cardiovascular disease.

Contraindications: Use of anticholinergic agents is contraindicated in patients with narrow angle glaucoma or prostatic hypertrophy. MAO-I use is contraindicated.

Advantages/Disadvantages: Diphenhydramine is not associated with dependance. It is less effective than benzodiazepines as a hypnotic. Use for insomnia should be limited to short periods.

Hydroxyzine (Atarax, Vistaril)

Category: Antihistamine, anxiolytic

Mechanism: Histamine receptor antagonist

Indications: Anxiety (short term treatment)

Preparations: 10, 25, 50, 100 mg tabs; 10 mg/5 ml syrup; 50 mg/ml solution (IM, not IV)

Hydroxyzine pamoate (Vistaril) - 25, 50, 100 mg caps; 25 mg/5 ml susp. (PO)

Dosage:

   Anxiety: 50-100 PO q 4-6 hrs.

   Acute agitation: 50-100 mg IM q 4-6 hrs.

Pharmacokinetics: Onset (fast), duration (short)

Side Effects: Dry mouth, dizziness, drowsiness, tremor, thickening of bronchial secretions, hypotension, decreased motor coordination, GI distress.

Interactions: Anticholinergics, MAO-I, Demerol, CNS depressants.

Major Safety Concerns: Driving may be contraindicated during early days of treatment. Use caution in patients with a history of urine retention, asthma, glaucoma, peptic ulcer disease, hyperthyroidism, hepatic or, cardiovascular disease.

Contraindications: Do not use in pregnancy or nursing (teratogenic effects in animal studies). MAO-I use is contraindicated.

Advantages/Disadvantages: Hydroxyzine is not associated with dependance. It is less effective than benzodiazepines for treatment of insomnia. Hydroxyzine use should be limited to 3 months.

Mood Stabilizers

Clinical Use of Mood Stabilizers

I. **Indications:** Mood stabilizers are indicated for the treatment of mania, depression, and mixed states associated with bipolar disorder, severe cyclothymia, and schizoaffective disorder. They are occasionally used in the treatment of impulse control disorders, severe personality disorders, and mental retardation.

II. **Categories**
    A. **Lithium** is the first-line treatment for bipolar disorder. It has antimanic and modest antidepressant properties. Concurrent use of an antidepressant is often required in the treatment of depressed patients.
    B. **Anticonvulsants** are useful in patients that have failed a drug trial of lithium. Anticonvulsants are more effective than lithium in the treatment of mania associated with rapid-cycling bipolar disorder. Two anticonvulsants are currently being utilized as mood stabilizers: Carbamazepine (Tegretol) and divalproex (Depakote). Their effectiveness as antidepressants is unproven.
    C. **Verapamil (Calan)** is an antihypertensive agent which has recently been demonstrated to have modest anti-mania properties. While lithium and the anticonvulsants are more effective, verapamil may be useful in patients who cannot tolerate the side effects of other mood stabilizers. Verapamil does not have antidepressant effects.

Carbamazepine (Tegretol)

Category: Anticonvulsant, mood stabilizer
Mechanism: Unknown. May be related to GABA level changes.
Indications: Approved for temporal lobe epilepsy and trigeminal neuralgia. Used clinically as antimanic agent in bipolar disorder and severe cyclothymia.
Preparations: 100, 200 mg caps; 100 mg/5 ml susp. (PO)
Dosage:
    Initially: 200 mg/day, then increase 200 mg every 2-4 days; not increase more than 200 mg/day until reach 800 mg daily dose
    Average dose: 600-1200 mg/day (divided doses)
    Dose range: 200-1600 mg/day (max. 2,200 mg/day)

Elderly: 200-1200 mg/day

Half-Life: Initially, 25-65 hrs. Reduced to 12-18 hrs. after several weeks of treatment.

Therapeutic Levels: 8-12 mcg/ml

Time to Therapeutic Effect: Antimanic effects occur in 2-4 weeks.

Side Effects: Sedation, blurred vision, nausea, GI distress, decreased TSH, ataxia, vertigo, dysarthria, rash, exfoliative dermatitis, delayed cardiac conduction, arrhythmias, hepatitis, aplastic anemia, agranulocytosis and, transient leukopenia. Most side effects occur at > 9 mcg/ml of carbamazepine. If significant **leukopenia** develops, then discontinue medication. Consider hematology consult if:

WBC < 3,000/mcL, neutrophils < 1,500/mcL, hematocrit. < 32 %, platelets < 100,000/mcL, reticulocytes < 0.3 %

Interactions:

  A. Antipsychotics - sedation, ataxia, dizziness
  B. Calcium channel blockers - increase CNS side effects
  C. Digitalis - bradycardia may result
  D. Lithium - both agents may decrease thyroid function and increase CNS side effects
  E. Theophylline - potentiate each other
  F. Divalproex sodium - displaces protein binding of carbamazepine
  G. Carbamazepine level may be increased by: cimetidine, diltiazem (not nifedipine), erythromycin, isoniazid, nicotinamide, valproic acid, propoxyphene, verapamil or, fluoxetine.
  H. Carbamazepine level may be decreased by: phenytoin, primidone, phenobarbital, TCAs or , theophylline.
  I. Carbamazepine may increase the level of clomipramine and phenytoin.
  J. Carbamazepine may decrease the effects of phenytoin, warfarin, ethosuximide, clonazepam, valproic acid, haloperidol, and, cyclic antidepressants

Major Safety Concerns: Severe blood dyscrasia (1:20,000) such as aplastic anemia and agranulocytosis may occur. Patients should contact their physician with the development of fever, sore throat, infection, bruising, bleeding, petechia. Use 1/3-1/2 dose in patients with hepatic disease.

Premedication lab screen: Check CBC with platelets, LFTs, serum electrolytes and BUN, UA and, ECG (patients over 40 or cardiac history).

Lab monitoring: Check CBC, LFTs, and blood level every 2 weeks for first 2 months, then every 4 months, then annually.

Contraindications: Carbamazepine is contraindicated in pregnancy and nursing, and in patients with glaucoma, cardiac, hepatic or, renal impairment. It is contraindicated in patients with a history of bone marrow suppression or

TCA allergic reactions. MAO-I use is contraindicated for 2 weeks before or after carbamazepine.

Advantages/Disadvantages: Carbamazepine may be more effective than lithium for **rapid cycling and dysphoric/mixed mania**. Side effects make carbamazepine a second line mood stabilizer (after lithium trial).

Lithium (Eskalith, Eskalith CR, Lithobid, Lithonate, Lithotabs)

Category: Mood stabilizer, antimanic

Mechanism: Unknown. Some suggest blockade of inositol-1-phosphatase or alteration of sodium channels.

Indications: Approved for treating manic symptoms of bipolar disorder. Used clinically for schizoaffective disorder, impulse control disorder, augmentation of antidepressant or antipsychotic, borderline personality disorder and, severe cyclothymia.

Preparations:

Rapid absorption - Eskalith caps (300 mg), Lithium carbonate caps and tabs (300 mg), Lithonate caps (300 mg), Lithotabs tabs (300 mg).

Slow release - Lithobid tabs (300 mg), Eskalith CR (450 mg).

Lithium citrate syrup: 8 mEq/5 ml (rapid absorption)

Dosage:

> Initially: Start with 300 mg PO bid/tid. Increase dose over 1-2 weeks to achieve therapeutic blood level of 0.8-1.2 mEq/L for acute mania.
>
> Following crisis resolution: Decrease dose to achieve maintenance blood level of 0.5-0.8 mEq/L. Continue at maintenance dose for 6-9 months.
>
> Average dose: 900-1200 mg/day (divided doses - bid/tid)
>
> Elderly or renal impairment: Start with 300 mg qd. Wide range of daily doses (100-900 mg).

Half-Life: 20 hrs.

Therapeutic Levels:

> Acute mania - 0.8-1.2 mEq/L
>
> Antimania maintenance - 0.5-0.8 mEq/L
>
> Check level at 5-7 days, 12 hrs. after last dose.
>
> Lithium level will be higher (approximately 30%) with slow release preparations.
>
> Mild-moderate toxicity at 1.5-2.0 mEq/L
>
> Severe toxicity at levels over 2.5 mEq/L

Time to Therapeutic Effect: Antimanic effect occurs in 2-6 weeks. Prophylactic effects develop in 2-3 months.

Side Effects: Most common: polyuria, increased thirst, GI distress, tremor, fatigue, cognitive impairment, weight gain. Also: headache, sedation, slurred speech, hypothyroidism, goiter, hyperglycemia, leukocytosis (benign, no treatment required) myocarditis, sinoatrial or atrioventricular block, T-wave flattening or inversion (benign, monitor, no treatment), syncope, hypotension, folliculitis, acne, rash, rarely exfoliative dermatitis (dermatology consult).

Treatment of Side Effects:

Diabetes insipidus - consider hydrochlorothiazide (50 mg/day) or amiloride (5-10 mg/day).

Edema - consider spironolactone 50 mg/day; monitor lithium.

Gastrointestinal distress - trial of slow release preparation or lower doses given more frequently.

Hypothyroidism - consider treatment with levothyroxine; follow TSH level.

Tremor - decrease dose, consider propranolol - starting with 10-20 mg bid, increasing to 20-60 mg/day. Also consider low dose clonazepam.

Interactions:

    A. Aminophylline - lithium excretion increased

    B. Antipsychotics - may increase neurotoxic effects of lithium

    C. Dietary sodium - too much may lower lithium level, too little may elevate lithium level

    D. Metronidazole - possible renal toxicity

    E. Potassium iodine - increases risk of goiter and hypothyroidism

    F. Lithium levels may be increased by: thiazides, amiloride, ethacrynic acid, furosemide, ibuprofen, tetracyclines, piroxicam, mefenamic acid, indomethacin, sulindac, tetracycline, triamterene, spironolactone, methyldopa, and metronidazole.

    G. Lithium levels may be decreased by: calcium channel blockers, valproate, theophylline, and diuretics.

Major Safety Concerns: Advise patients to maintain adequate fluid intake. Sweating and dehydration increases lithium level and risk of toxicity. Patients should attempt to discontinue lithium 1-2 months prior to planned conception.

Initial laboratory screen: Check CBC, BUN, serum creatinine, thyroid function panel, urinalysis, HCG, serum electrolytes and fasting glucose, ECG

Laboratory monitoring: Check renal function (serum creatinine, urine specific gravity) every 3-6 months. Check TSH every six months.

Lithium monitoring: Check lithium level weekly for first month, then biweekly for 2-3 months, then every 1-2 months. Check lithium level 3-4 times per year after 1 year.

Overdose/intoxication signs: Nausea, vomiting, renal failure, confusion, incoordination, concentration problems, dysarthria, tremor, ataxia, delirium, seizure, coma.

Contraindications: Lithium use is contraindicated in pregnancy (**teratogenic** effects), breast-feeding, or patients with history of myocardial infarction. Use caution in patients with hypothyroidism and, cardiovascular or renal impairment.

Advantages/Disadvantages: Lithium is useful in several disorders displaying mood instability and depression. Prophylaxis of recurrent manic episodes may improve long term prognosis of bipolar disorder by reducing cycle frequency and by maintaining responsiveness to lithium. Major compliance problems occur in bipolar disorder due to loss of manic excitement and frequent side effects.

Valproic Acid (Depakene), Divalproex (Depakote)

Category: Anticonvulsant, antimanic
Mechanism: Unknown. May involve GABA level changes.
Indications: Divalproex approved as treatment for mania. Both agents used clinically for bipolar disorder.
Preparations:
Valproic acid (generic) - 250 mg caps
Valproic acid (Depakene) - 250 mg caps, 250 mg/5 ml syrup
Divalproex sodium (Depakote) - delayed release - 125, 250, 500 mg tabs; 125 mg sprinkle caps (earlier onset, lower peak than tablets)
Dosage:
    Initially: 250 mg on first day, then increase 250 mg every 3 days
    Average dose: 1000-1500 mg/day (tid dosing)
    Dose range: 250-2000 mg/day (divided doses)
    Elderly: 250-100 mg/day
Half-Life: 8-10 hrs.
Therapeutic Levels: 50-125 mcg/ml
Time to Therapeutic Effect: 2-4 weeks for antimanic effects
Side Effects: Most common - sedation, nausea, vomiting; also - CNS depression, tremor, hyperammonemia, GI upset, weight gain, ataxia, headache, hair loss, rash, clotting abnormalities, rare pancreatitis and hepatitis, **transient transaminase elevation** (most resolve in 6 months).
Interactions:
    A. Anticoagulants - potentiation
    B. Antipsychotics - levels of both agents may be increased, sedation and EPS may increase
    C. Aspirin - potentiates anticoagulation
    D. Carbamazepine - level increased by protein displacement

   E. CNS depressants (e.g., alcohol, phenobarbital) - potentiate depression

   F. Lithium - increased tremor

   G. Thyroid function test - false abnormalities

   H. Warfarin - potentiate anticoagulation

   I. Divalproex sodium level may be increased by antipsychotics, cimetidine, fluoxetine, amitriptyline and, diazepam.

Major Safety Concerns: Use caution in patients with a history of liver disorder or renal disease. Complicated interactions with other anticonvulsants may warrant neurology consult for combination treatment.

Hepatic failure, when present, usually in first 6 months, and may be preceded by weakness, facial edema, anorexia, vomiting or, jaundice.

Premedication lab screen: LFTs, CBC, PT/PTT

Follow-up lab monitoring: Frequent LFTs over first 6 months.

Contraindications: Divalproex sodium is contraindicated in patients with liver disease or dysfunction, pregnancy or nursing (reports of **teratogenic** effects in humans).

Advantages/Disadvantages: Divalproex sodium is approved for treatment of mania (unlike carbamazepine). It is effective against mania and, possibly, depression of bipolar disorder but is generally regarded as a second-line treatment (after lithium trial). Divalproex sodium is more effective than lithium in the treatment of rapid cycling and dysphoric mania bipolar disorder. Divalproex sodium's short half life warrants a tid dosing schedule.

Verapamil (Calan, Isoptin, Verelan)

Category: Antihypertensive agent, mood stabilizer

Mechanism: Calcium ion influx inhibitor. Increase synaptic calcium levels.

Indications: Approved for hypertension, angina, arrhythmias. Used clinically as antimanic for treatment-refractory bipolar disorder.

Preparations: 40, 80, 120 mg tabs; slow release form (Calan SR) - 120, 180, 240 mg tabs

Dosage:
   Initially: 40 mg tid, then increase over 1 week to 80-120 mg tid
   Dose range: 240-440 mg/day (divided doses)
   Elderly: Lower doses required

Half-Life: 3-7 hrs. for first dose; 4-12 hrs. after multiple doses.

Therapeutic Levels: Not established

Side Effects: Hypotension, bradycardia, AV block, nausea, diarrhea, constipation, fatigue, headache, dizziness, exacerbation of

Interactions:
  A. Antipsychotics - may increase extrapyramidal symptoms.
  B. Carbamazepine - verapamil increases carbamazepine level (decrease carbamazepine dose by one half when combining with verapamil); neurotoxicity may result.
  C. Fluoxetine - increase verapamil; edema, headache.
  D. Lithium - neurotoxicity, dyskinesia, bradycardia; verapamil may also decrease lithium level.
  E. Tagamet - may increase verapamil level.

Major Safety Concerns: Monitor heart rate, blood pressure, ECG (especially if history of cardiac disease). Avoid use during pregnancy and lactation. Decrease dose in patients with hepatic disease. Use caution in patients with a history of conduction defects.

Contraindications: Verapamil is contraindicated in patients with severe left ventricular dysfunction, hypotension, sick sinus syndrome, second or third degree AV block, atrial flutter or fibrillation. Do not use verapamil with beta blockers, hypotensive medications or, antiarrhythmics.

Advantages/Disadvantages: Verapamil is a useful option in patients with bipolar disorder who cannot tolerate or do not respond to lithium, divalproex sodium, or carbamazepine. No specific pretreatment laboratory tests are required.

Stimulants

Clinical Use of Stimulants

I. **Indications**
   A. Psychostimulants, or centrally acting stimulants, have been approved for the treatment of narcolepsy and attention deficit hyperactivity disorder (ADHD). These agents improve concentration.
   B. Stimulants are also used clinically for the diagnosis and treatment of specific types of depression as described below.

II. **Categories**
   A. Amphetamine and amphetamine-like agents include dextroamphetamine (Dexadrine) and methylphenidate (Ritalin). Use of these agents has been controversial in some circumstances, particularly when diagnosis is unclear.
   B. The only nonamphetamine-like stimulant currently being used to treat ADHD is pemoline (Cylert). Both the effectiveness and abuse potential are lesser for pemoline than for amphetamine-like agents.

Dextroamphetamine (Dexedrine)

Category: Amphetamine
Mechanism: Dopamine release at synapse, catecholamine reuptake inhibition and, MAO-I inhibition.
Indications: Approved for attention deficit disorder and narcolepsy. Used clinically for diagnosis and short term treatment of depression in the medically ill. Also, used for augmentation of partial response to antidepressant medication.
Preparations:
Dextroamphetamine sulfate (Dexedrine) - 5 mg tabs
Dexedrine Spansule (sustained release) - 5, 10, 15 mg caps
Dosage:
   Attention Deficit/hyperactivity Disorder (ADHD): Initially 2.5 mg/day. Gradually increase to 5-20 mg/day in divided doses.
   Child dose range: 2.5-40 mg/day (max. 0.5 mg/kg). Morning administration.
   Adult dose range: 2.5-20 mg/day (max. 40 mg/day).

Depression (medically ill): 15 mg/day (short term).

Antidepressant augmentation: 5-20 mg/day.

Half Life: 6 hrs.

Side Effects: CNS stimulation, euphoria (short term), anxiety, irritability, hypertension, dry mouth, anorexia, insomnia, palpitations, urticaria, psychosis, depression, GI distress, decreased appetite (short term), movement disorders.

Interactions:

1. Antihypertensives - decreases hypotensive effects
2. Antidepressants - augmentation of antidepressant effects
3. Beta adrenergic blockers - inhibit action
4. MAO-I - possible hypertensive crisis
5. Decrease metabolism and increase level of: Tricyclic and tetracyclic antidepressants, warfarin, phenytoin, phenobarbital, primidone, phenylbutazone.

Major Safety Concerns: Cardiovascular side effects warrant premedication and follow-up monitoring of blood pressure and ECG. Decrease dose in patients with renal or hepatic disease. Dextroamphetamine may exacerbate glaucoma, cardiovascular disease, hyperthyroidism or, seizure disorder. Long term or high dose use of stimulants may induce psychosis. Monitor patients for dependence and abuse.

Contraindications: Amphetamines are contraindicated in symptomatic cardiovascular disease, moderate to severe hypertension, advanced arteriosclerosis and, hyperthyroidism. MAO-I use is contraindicated within 2 weeks of dextroamphetamine. Amphetamines are not recommended for children under 3 years of age. Do not use amphetamines with agitated patients. Avoid stimulant use in patients with a history of substance abuse and those who are pregnant or nursing (possible teratogen). Do not use amphetamines in patients with tic movement disorders or family history of Tourette's Syndrome (consider use of desipramine).

Advantages/Disadvantages: Tolerance develops to euphoria but not cognitive benefits to attention deficit disorder. Amphetamines lead to rapid response of depression (1-2 days). Antidepressant effects are brief for many patients (2-4 weeks). Short half life requires tid dosing.

Methylphenidate (Ritalin, Ritalin SR)

Category: CNS stimulant (similar structure to amphetamine)
Mechanism: Releases catecholamine at synapse, decreases dopamine reuptake and, inhibits MAO-I.
Indications: Approved for attention deficit disorder and narcolepsy. Used clinically for short term treatment of depression in medically ill. Also, used for augmentation of partial response to antidepressant agent.
Preparations: 5, 10, 20 mg tabs; sustained release - 20 mg tabs
Dosage:

> Attention Deficit/Hyperactivity Disorder (ADHD): Initiate with 5 mg bid (AM doses). Increase by 5 mg bid each week.
>
> Child range: 10-60 mg/day (max. 0.5 mg/kg)
>
> Adult range: 10-60 mg/day (max. 60-80 mg/day)
>
> Depression (medically ill): 15 mg/day (short term).
>
> Augmentation of antidepressant - 10-40 mg/day

Half Life: 2-3 hrs.
Side Effects: CNS stimulation, euphoria (short term), anxiety, irritability, hypertension, dry mouth, anorexia, insomnia, palpitations, urticaria, psychosis, depression, GI distress, decreased appetite (short term), movement disorders.
Interactions:

1. Antihypertensives - decreases hypotensive effects
2. Antidepressants - augmentation of antidepressant effects
3. MAO-I - hypertensive crisis may result
4. Methylphenidate decreases metabolism and increases level of: Tricyclic and tetracyclic antidepressants, warfarin, phenytoin, phenobarbital, primidone and, phenylbutazone.

Major Safety Concerns: Cardiovascular side effects warrant monitoring of blood pressure. Decrease dose in patients with renal or hepatic disease. Methylphenidate may exacerbate glaucoma, cardiovascular disease, hyperthyroidism or, seizure disorder. Dependence and abuse are possible. Periodic CBC and liver function tests are advised.
Contraindications: Methylphenidate is contraindicated in patients with symptomatic cardiovascular disease, moderate to severe hypertension, advanced arteriosclerosis and, hyperthyroidism. It is not recommended for children under 6 years of age or patients in an agitated state. MAO-I use is contraindicated within 2 weeks of methylphenidate. Avoid use of stimulants in patients with a history of substance abuse. Methylphenidate is not recommended in patients with tic movement disorders or family history of Tourette's Syndrome (consider use of desipramine).
Advantages/Disadvantages: Tolerance   develops   to   euphoria   of

methylphenidate but cognitive benefits to attention deficit disorder are not diminished. Amphetamine-like agents lead to rapid clinical response. Antidepressant effects are brief (2-4 weeks for most patients). Short half life requires tid/qid dosing.

Pemoline (Cylert)

Category: CNS stimulant (unrelated to amphetamine)
Mechanism: Potentiates catecholamines
Indications: Attention deficit disorder
Preparations: 18.75, 37.5, 75 mg tabs; 37.5 chewable tabs
Dosage:
> Attention Deficit/hyperactivity Disorder (ADHD): Initially, 18.75-37.5 mg (child and adult). Increase weekly by 18.75-37.5 mg/day.
> Child dose range - 37.5-112.5 mg/day (single dose/day)
> Adult dose range - limited data available; some recommend 56.25-75 mg/day (max. 112.5 mg/day)

Half Life: 12 hrs.
Side Effects: CNS stimulation, anorexia (short term), insomnia, headache, rash, GI upset, hepatitis, jaundice, decrease seizure threshold, motor tics, possible growth suppression.
Interactions: Limited data is available. Increases excitatory effects of other CNS stimulants.
Major Safety Concern: Pemoline is associated with a risk of reversible liver abnormalities and jaundice. Monitor liver function tests. Avoid pemoline use in severe renal impairment.
Contraindications: Pemoline is contraindicated in patients with impaired renal function. It is not recommended for children under 6 years of age or patients with a family history of tic disorder (consider use of desipramine).
Advantages/Disadvantages: Pemoline has less effect on blood pressure and heart rate than other stimulants. It has lower abuse potential but, less effectiveness than dextroamphetamine and methylphenidate. Pemoline has a slower onset of therapeutic effect than other stimulants (3-4 weeks).

Substance Abuse

Management of Substance Abuse

I. **Indications:** Although the foundation for treatment of substance abuse continues to be psychotherapy and support group activities, medications may be used as adjuncts to assist patients in the early weeks and months of recovery.

II. **Categories**
   A. **Alcohol abuse prevention**
      1. Reduction of alcohol craving has been reported with use of naltrexone (ReVia). Benefits are very modest.
      2. Deterrence of alcohol use can be facilitated with the use of disulfiram (Antabuse). Used as directed, disulfiram is highly effective in preventing alcohol use.
   B. **Alcohol withdrawal seizure prophylaxis:** Prevention of alcohol withdrawal seizures can be accomplished by short term use of benzodiazepines. Three to five days of diazepam (Valium) use provides effective prevention. Other benzodiazepines are also useful (see benzodiazepine section).
   C. **Opioid abuse prevention:** Naltrexone (ReVia) reduces opioid craving in some individuals.
   D. **Opioid withdrawal treatment:** Opioid agonists may be used in the treatment of severe opioid dependence. Use of methadone (Dolophine) reduces opioid craving and lessens physical aspects of withdrawal, but remains a controversial treatment method. Clonidine (Catapres) may be used to lessen physiologic manifestations of opioid withdrawal.

Clonidine (Catapres, Catapres-TTS)

Category: Antihypertensive agent
Mechanism: Alpha 2 adrenergic receptor agonist
Indications: Approved for hypertension. Used clinically for opioid withdrawal and Tourette's Syndrome.
Preparations: 0.1, 0.2, 0.3 mg tabs; Clonidine TTS patch - 2.5 mg/ 3.5 cm (0.1 mg/day), 5.0 mg/ 7.0 cm, 7.5 mg/ 10.5 cm (0.3 mg/day)
Dosage:

Methadone withdrawal: 0.15 mg bid

Opiate withdrawal: 0.1-0.3 q 6-8 hrs. prn autonomic signs (max. 2.5/day). Establish 24 hr. requirement, then taper by 0.1 mg/day.

Tourette's syndrome (child): Start with 0.05 mg/day. Gradually increase to range of 0.05-0.3 mg/day (divided doses) for 3 month trial.

Half Life: 12-16 hrs.

Side Effects: Hypotension, sedation, dizziness, fatigue, dry mouth, nausea, constipation, sexual dysfunction, insomnia, anxiety, depression, photophobia, rash, weight gain.

Interactions:

A. Beta blockers - increase rebound hypertension

B. CNS depressants - potentiate depression

C. Diuretics - hypotension may occur

D. TCAs - inhibit hypotensive effect of clonidine

Major Safety Concerns: Taper clonidine dose when discontinuing use (rebound effects 20 hours after last dose). Use caution in patients with a history of cardiac disease, Raynaud's Syndrome, or depression. Adjust dose in patients with renal impairment.

Contraindications: Avoid use of clonidine if blood pressure is less than 90/60.

Advantages/Disadvantages: Clonidine reduces the autonomic signs of opioid withdrawal but does not reduce subjective symptoms. Clonidine may be used alone for detoxification but usually follows methadone taper.

Disulfiram (Antabuse)

Category: Alcohol abuse deterrent

Mechanism: Aldehyde dehydrogenase inhibitor. Leads to elevated levels of acetaldehyde.

Indications: Alcohol dependence

Preparations: 250, 500 mg tabs

Dosage: Alcohol abuse deterrent: 250-500 mg qd

Half Life: 60-120 hrs.

Side Effects: Fatigue, headaches, impotence, acne, rash, irritability, insomnia, confusion, hepatitis. less commonly: peripheral neuropathy, blood dyscrasias, delirium, psychosis.

If alcohol consumed: headache, nausea, vomiting, pallor, thirst, diaphoresis, chest pain, anxiety, blurred vision, respiratory depression, arrhythmias, heart failure, seizure, death.

Interactions:

A. Alcohol - fatal reaction is possible (described above)
B. CNS depressants - potentiates depression
C. Isoniazid - behavioral changes possible
D. Metronidazole - may precipitate psychosis
E. Theophylline - potentiates actions of theophylline
F. Tricyclic antidepressants - organic brain syndrome may develop
G. Disulfiram may increase levels of: diazepam, paraldehyde, phenytoin, caffeine, tricyclic antidepressants, anticoagulants, barbiturates or, anticoagulants.

Major Safety Concerns: A risk of severe alcohol reaction remains for two weeks after last dose of disulfiram. Use caution in patients with a history of renal or hepatic disease, CNS disorder, hypothyroidism or, over age 50. Premedication CBC and liver function tests are recommended. Periodic monitoring of liver function tests is advised. Warn patients about dietary and over the counter preparations that may contain alcohol. Patients should get a drug alert identification card or tag identifying their use of disulfiram.

Contraindications: Disulfiram is contraindicated in patients with severe cardiovascular or pulmonary disease. Alcohol use within 14 days of this medication is contraindicated.

Advantages/Disadvantages: Brief use of disulfiram (e.g.,1-3 months) may help otherwise weakly motivated patients initiate pattern of sobriety. Disulfiram should be used in conjunction with a recovery program. Risk of fatality has limited its clinical use.

Methadone (Dolophine)

Category: Synthetic opioid
Mechanism: Mu opioid receptor agonist
Indications: Detoxification and maintenance treatment of opioid addiction.
Preparations: 5, 10, 40 mg tabs; 5 mg/ 5 ml soln., 10 mg/ 5 ml soln., 10 mg/ ml soln. (PO); 10 mg/ml soln. (IV, IM)
Dosage:
> Detoxification: Short term use (3-30 days). Initially, 10-20 mg prn signs of withdrawal. Increase by 5 mg prn for 24 hrs. Maximum use of 20 mg/ 12 hrs.(unless severe dependence). Then, calculate 24 hr. dose and decrease by 5 mg/day until reaching 15 mg/day. Then, decrease by 5 mg qOD.
> Maintenance: Use lowest tolerable dose.

Half Life: 24-36 hrs.
Side Effects: Sedation, insomnia, dependence, dizziness, euphoria,

sweating, agitation, seizure, delirium, colic, nausea, vomiting, constipation, urine retention, flushing, rash, menstrual changes, respiratory depression.

Interactions: Cautious use with CNS depressants   (e.g.,meperidine, fentanyl), low potency antipsychotics, tricyclic and tetracyclic antidepressants, and MAO-Is. Methadone level is decreased by carbamazepine, phenobarbital, rifampin, and phenytoin.

Major Safety Concerns: Tolerance to euphoric effects may lead to overdose. Respiratory depression may occur with overdose. Use caution in patients with a history of respiratory disease, hepatic or renal abnormalities, seizure disorder or, head injury. Warn patients about driving and other safety hazards of sedation. MAO-I use is contraindicated within 14 days of methadone.

Advantages/Disadvantages: Successful detoxification and rehabilitation may reduce risk of HIV infection. Prolonged methadone use may substitute one addiction for another. Methadone use longer than 3 weeks may be limited to specialized treatment programs.

Psychiatric Side Effect Management

Management of Psychotherapeutic Agent Side Effects

I. **Indications:** Medication may be used for the treatment of drug-induced side effects when other attempts to manage side effects have failed. Initial steps to manage side effects should include reducing the dosage (if therapeutic effect can be maintained) and changing class of drug (e.g., tricyclic antidepressant to serotonin specific reuptake inhibitor). Some medication side effects, such as neuroleptic malignant syndrome, requires immediate medication and supportive measures.

II. **Categories**
    A. **Neuroleptic malignant syndrome** treatments may include a dopamine agonist such as amantadine (Symmetrel) and a muscle relaxant such as dantrolene (Dantrium).
    B. **Extrapyramidal symptoms**, associated with typical antipsychotics, may be treated with anticholinergic agents such as diphenhydramine (Benadryl) or benztropine (Cogentin).
    C. **Tremors**, associated with lithium use, may be treated with anticholinergic agents, beta adrenergic blockers or, benzodiazepines.
    D. **Sexual dysfunction**, associated with serotonin antagonists, may be treated with antihistamines such as cyproheptadine (Periactin) or sympathomimetics such as yohimbine (Yocon).

Amantadine (Symmetrel)

Category: Antiparkinsonian agent
Mechanism: Dopamine agonist
Indications: Neuroleptic induced extrapyramidal symptoms (EPS)
Preparations: 100 mg caps; 50 mg/ 5 ml syrup
Dosage:
    Chronic EPS: 100 mg tid (max. 400 mg/day)
Half Life: 10-25 hrs.
Side Effects: Nausea, dry mouth, blurred vision, constipation, anorexia, hypotension, dizziness, anxiety, tremor, insomnia, irritability, impaired concentration, psychosis, seizure.

Interactions:

- **A.** Anticholinergics - potentiation
- **B.** CNS stimulants - irritability, seizure, arrhythmia
- **C.** Thiazides - may increase level of amantadine
- **D.** Sympathomimetics - potentiation

Major Safety Concerns: Neuroleptic malignant syndrome has been reported with dose reduction or discontinuation of amantadine. Reduce dose in elderly. Use caution in patients with a history of edema or congestive heart failure. Perform trial off amantadine after 4 weeks to assess the need for continued use. Taper drug when discontinuing use.

Contraindications: Avoid amantadine use in pregnancy and lactation (embryotoxic and teratogenic in animals). Alcohol should not be used with this medication. Amantadine use is contraindicated in patients with a history of renal disease or seizure.

Advantages/Disadvantages: Amantadine is associated with less memory impairment than anticholinergics. It is useful when anticholinergics must be avoided. Amantadine is less effective than anticholinergics in treatment of acute dystonias.

Atenolol (Tenormin)

Category: Antihypertensive agent

Mechanism: Beta-1 adrenergic receptor blockade

Indications: Approved for hypertension and angina. Used clinically for lithium induced tremor, neuroleptic induced akathisia, and somatic signs of anxiety (e.g., social phobia).

Preparations: 25, 50, 100 mg tabs

Dosage:

> Tremor, akathisia, or anxiety: Initially, 50 mg/day (max. 100 mg/day)
> Elderly: 25-100 mg/day

Half Life: 6-9 hrs.

Side Effects: Hypotension, bradycardia, arrhythmia, nausea/ vomiting, diarrhea, dizziness, fatigue, insomnia, depression, sexual dysfunction, AV node heart block, inhibit insulin release (increases blood sugar).

Interactions:

- **A.** Anticonvulsants - altered metabolism; monitor levels
- **B.** Antipsychotics - altered metabolism; monitor levels
- **C.** Barbiturates - decreased levels of atenolol
- **D.** Calcium channel blockers - conduction abnormalities may develop
- **E.** Insulin and oral hypoglycemics - glucose level changes

F. MAO-I - possible hypertensive crisis(see MAOI section)

Major Safety Concerns: Taper dose of atenolol when discontinuing use. Use caution in patients with renal/ hepatic disorder. See contraindications.

Contraindications: Atenolol is contraindicated in patients with pulmonary disease (e.g., **asthma**), diabetes, hyperthyroidism, angina, heart block, overt congestive heart failure, peripheral vascular disease, pregnancy and lactation (fetal injury in animals).

Advantages/Disadvantages: Single daily dosing is possible. Atenolol lacks the dependence associated with benzodiazepine treatment of anxiety or tremor.

Benztropine (Cogentin)

Category: Antiparkinsonian agent
Mechanism: Muscarinic cholinergic receptor antagonist
Indications: Neuroleptic induced extrapyramidal symptoms (EPS)
Preparations: 0.5, 1, 2 mg tabs; 1 mg/ml soln. (IV, IM)
Dosage:
  Acute dystonia: 1-2 mg IM (max. 6 mg/day)
  Chronic EPS: 1-2 mg PO bid/tid
Side Effects: Drowsiness, dry mouth, blurred vision, nausea, weakness, confusion, constipation, urine retention, sedation, drowsiness, depression, psychosis.
Interactions:
  A. Antacids - delay concurrent use of benztropine for 1 hour
  B. Anticholinergics (e.g., low potency neuroleptics, tricyclics, over-the-counter sleep preparations) - anticholinergic intoxication may develop
  C. CNS depressants - potentiation of depression
Major Safety Concerns: Sedative effect may impair driving and performance of potentially hazardous tasks. Avoid using this medication with low potency neuroleptics (excess anticholinergic effects). Advise patients to avoid dehydration and hyperthermia during hot weather. Perform trial off benztropine in 4 weeks to determine if continued use is necessary. Taper medication off over 2 weeks.
Contraindications: Avoid benztropine use in glaucoma, prostatic hypertrophy, myasthenia gravis, duodenal or pyloric obstruction.
Advantages/Disadvantages: Prophylactic use of benztropine may prevent uncomfortable side effects of antipsychotics, especially with high potency agents in young males. Benztropine is the most widely used agent for EPS. IV and IM use are equally effective - use the IM route. Benztropine is the **least**

sedating of the anticholinergic agents. Anticholinergic agents are less effective than propranolol or benzodiazepines in the treatment of akathisia.

Biperiden (Akineton)

Category: Antiparkinsonian agent
Mechanism: Muscarinic cholinergic receptor antagonist
Indications: Neuroleptic induced extrapyramidal symptoms (EPS)
Preparations: 2 mg tabs; 5 mg/ml (IV, IM)
Dosage:

Acute dystonia: 2 mg IM. Repeat in 20 minutes, if needed.

Chronic EPS: 2 mg PO bid/tid (max. 6 mg/day)

Side Effects: Drowsiness, dry mouth, blurred vision, nausea, weakness, confusion, constipation, urine retention, sedation, drowsiness, depression, psychosis.

Interactions:

   A. Antacids - delay concurrent use of biperiden for 1 hour
   B. Anticholinergics (e.g., low potency neuroleptics, tricyclics, over the counter sleep preparations) - anticholinergic intoxication may develop
   C. CNS depressants - potentiation of depression

Major Safety Concerns: Sedative effect may impair driving and performance of potentially hazardous tasks. Avoid using this medication with low potency neuroleptics (excess anticholinergic effects). Advise patients to avoid dehydration and hyperthermia during hot weather. Perform trial off biperiden in 4 weeks to determine if continued use is necessary. Taper medication over 2 weeks.

Contraindications: Avoid biperiden use in glaucoma, prostatic hypertrophy, myasthenia gravis, duodenal or pyloric obstruction.

Advantages/Disadvantages: Prophylactic use of biperiden may prevent uncomfortable side effects of antipsychotics, especially with high potency agents in young males. Anticholinergic agents are less effective than propranolol or benzodiazepines in the treatment of akathisia.

Dantrolene (Dantrium)

Category: Muscle relaxant, anti-hyperthermia agent
Mechanism: Impairs calcium release from sarcoplasmic reticulum.
Indications: Approved for chronic spasticity and, prevention and treatment of hyperthermia. Used clinically to treat neuroleptic malignant syndrome.
Preparations: 25, 50, 100 mg caps; 20 mg powder
Dosage:
> Neuroleptic malignant syndrome: 1 mg/kg PO qid or 1-5 mg/kg IV. Repeat every 5 minutes, as needed (max. 10 mg/kg/day).

Half Life: 9 hrs.
Side Effects: Depression, weakness, drowsiness, slurred speech, dizziness, confusion, nausea, GI upset, hepatitis with long term use.
Interactions:
>   A. Calcium channel blockers - verapamil is associated with rare reports of cardiovascular collapse
>   B. CNS depressants - potentiation of depression
>   C. Estrogen - possible hepatotoxicity over age 35.

Major Safety Concerns: Dantrolene may cause hepatotoxicity. Overt hepatitis is most often seen after 3 months of treatment. Monitor LFTs. Use caution in patients with respiratory or cardiac disease, or history of hepatic disease.
Contraindications: Dantrolene is contraindicated in patients with liver disease or elevation of liver enzymes.
Disadvantage: Tissue necrosis may occur with extravasation of IV fluid.

Procyclidine (Kemadrin)

Category: Antiparkinsonian agent, antispasmodic agent
Mechanism: Muscarinic cholinergic receptor antagonist
Indications: Neuroleptic induced extrapyramidal symptoms (EPS)
Preparations: 5 mg tabs
Dosage: Chronic EPS: Initially, 2.5 mg tid. Increase to 5 mg tid as needed (max. 20 mg/day).
Side Effects: Drowsiness, dry mouth, blurred vision, nausea, weakness, confusion, constipation, urine retention, sedation, drowsiness, depression, psychosis.
Interactions:
>   A. Antacids - delay concurrent use of procyclidine for 1 hour

    B. Anticholinergics (e.g., low potency neuroleptics, tricyclics, over the counter preparations) - possible anticholinergic intoxication

    C. CNS depressants - potentiation of depression

Major Safety Concerns: Sedative effect may impair driving and performance of potentially hazardous tasks. Avoid using this medication with low potency neuroleptics (excess anticholinergic effects). Advise patients to avoid dehydration and hyperthermia during hot weather. Perform trial off procyclidine in 4 weeks to determine if continued use is necessary. Taper medication off over 2 weeks.

Contraindications: Avoid procyclidine use in glaucoma, prostatic hypertrophy, myasthenia gravis, duodenal or pyloric obstruction.

Advantages/Disadvantages: Prophylactic use of procyclidine may prevent uncomfortable side effects of antipsychotics, especially with high potency agents in young males. Anticholinergic agents are less effective than propranolol or benzodiazepines in the treatment of akathisia.

Propranolol (Inderal)

Category: Antihypertensive agent

Mechanism: Beta-1 and beta-2 adrenergic receptor blockade

Indications: Approved for hypertension, angina, and migraine headaches. Used clinically for lithium induced tremor, acute neuroleptic induced akathisia, and somatic signs of anxiety (e.g., social phobia).

Preparations: 10, 20, 40, 80 mg tabs; Inderal-LA (long acting) - 60, 80, 120 mg caps

Dosage:

    Initially: 10 mg tid, then increase by 20 mg/day.

    Lithium tremor: 60-420 mg/day

    Social phobia: 10-40 mg 30 minutes prior to performance

    Elderly: 40-160 mg/day

Half Life: 3-6 hrs. (short acting form)

Side Effects: Hypotension, bradycardia, arrhythmia, nausea/ vomiting, diarrhea, dizziness, fatigue, insomnia, depression, sexual dysfunction, AV node heart block, inhibit insulin release (increase blood sugar).

Interactions:

    A. Anticonvulsants - altered metabolism; monitor levels

    B. Antipsychotics - altered metabolism; monitor levels

    C. Barbiturates - decreased levels of atenolol

    D. Calcium channel blockers - possible conduction abnormalities

    E. Cimetidine - increases level of propranolol

    F. Insulin and oral hypoglycemics - glucose level changes
    G. MAO-I - possible hypertensive crisis
    H. Thyroxine - lower T3

Major Safety Concerns: Taper dose of propranolol when discontinuing use (e.g., 20 mg every 3 days). Use caution in patients with a history of renal or hepatic disorder.

Contraindications: Propranolol is contraindicated in patients with a history of pulmonary disease (e.g., **asthma**), diabetes, hyperthyroidism, angina, heart block, heart failure or, peripheral vascular disease. Avoid use of this medication in pregnancy and lactation (fetal injury in animals).

Advantages/Disadvantages: Daily dosing is possible with LA form. Propranolol lacks the dependence associated with benzodiazepine treatment of anxiety or akathisia.

Trihexyphenidyl (Artane)

Category: Antiparkinsonian agent
Mechanism: Muscarinic cholinergic receptor antagonist
Indications: Neuroleptic induced extrapyramidal symptoms (EPS)
Preparations: 2, 5 mg tabs, 5 mg caps
Dosage:
Initially: 1 mg qd, then increase to 2 mg bid-qid (max. 15 mg/day)
Side Effects: Drowsiness, dry mouth, blurred vision, nausea, weakness, confusion, constipation, urine retention, sedation, drowsiness, depression, psychosis.
Interactions:
    A. Antacids - delay concurrent use of trihexyphenidyl for 1 hour
    B. Anticholinergics (e.g., low potency neuroleptics, tricyclics, over the counter sleep preparations) - anticholinergic intoxication may develop
    C. CNS depressants - potentiation of depression

Major Safety Concerns: Sedative effect may impair driving and performance of potentially hazardous tasks. Avoid using this medication with low potency neuroleptics (excess anticholinergic effects). Advise patients to avoid dehydration and hyperthermia during hot weather. Perform trial off trihexyphenidyl in 4 weeks to determine if continued use is necessary. Taper medication off over 2 weeks.

Contraindications: Avoid trihexyphenidyl use in glaucoma, prostatic hypertrophy, myasthenia gravis, duodenal or pyloric obstruction.

Advantages/Disadvantages: Prophylactic use of trihexyphenidyl may prevent uncomfortable side effects of antipsychotics, especially with high potency agents in young males. Anticholinergic agents are less effective than propranolol or benzodiazepines in the treatment of akathisia. Trihexyphenidyl is the most **stimulating** of the anticholinergic agents.

Index